THE PSYCHOTHERAPIST'S ESSENTIAL GUIDE TO THE BRAIN

THE PSYCHOTHERAPIST'S ESSENTIAL GUIDE TO THE BRAIN

Matthew Dahlitz

Edited by Geoff Hall

DAHLITZ MEDIA ☰

Dahlitz Media
Brisbane, Australia

Note to Readers: This book is intended as general information for mental health professionals and is not an appropriate substitute for training or clinical supervision. Neuroscience is a rapidly advancing field and neither the publisher nor the author can guarantee the complete accuracy or currency of the information herein. Clinical application of any information or techniques, including the contents of this book, should be undertaken only after certified training and appropriate supervision.

Chapters in this edition have previously been published in *The Neuropsychotherapist*.

For information about content reproduction write to: Permissions, The Neuropsychotherapist, PO Box 1030, Park Ridge, QLD, 4125, Australia.
Alternatively email editor@neuropsychotherapist.com

Author: Matthew Dahlitz
Editor: Geoff Hall

Cover image: EpicStockMedia/Bigstock.com

Title: The Psychotherapist's Essential Guide To The Brain.

ISBN-13: 978-0-9944080-1-3 (paperback)
ISBN-10: 0-9944080-1-3

1. Psychotherapy. 2. Brain. 3. Neuroscience. 4. Psychology. 5. Biopsychology.

Dahlitz Media
PO Box 1030
Park Ridge,
Queensland, 4125
AUSTRALIA

Printed in the United States of America

NEUROPSYCHOTHERAPIST.COM

To Shera
who has been long-suffering
in lending me to the insatiable desire
to know more.

CONTENTS

INTRODUCTION 1

An overview of major brain divisions, the complexity of networks and functions of neurons.

DEEP SYSTEMS 17

The function of the limbic system including the thalamus, amygdala, hippocampus and hypothalamus.

THE NEOCORTEX 27

Major divisions and functions of the neocortex. In particular the function of the prefrontal cortex in cognition and higher order processing.

NEUROCHEMICALS 35

An overview of the types and functions of neurotransmitters utilized by the brain including the neurochemistry of stress.

EPIGENETICS 41

How environmental factors influence gene expression both within and through heritable changes in DNA that can be transient or lifelong.

MOTIVATION 45

How the striatum and the belief that we have some control over our environment motivates us.

MIRROR NEURONS 49

Mirror neurons respond to acts that are perceived to carry purpose or intention and form an important part of learning and being empathic.

PREFACE

In February 2016, *The Neuropsychotherapist*, a magazine devoted to informing mental health professionals about the neuroscience of psychotherapy, introduced a regular column on the brain for the practising clinician. The column proved popular because it interpreted relevant facts from a large body of technical knowledge in language accessible to the non-scientist. In view of the positive readership response, it was decided to compile all instalments of The Psychotherapist's Essential Guide to the Brain together with new material into a stand-alone volume that might become a handy addition to the psychotherapist's bookshelf.

Why learn about the brain? Surely a therapist has a range of therapies and techniques at his or her disposal that can be effectively implemented without a degree in neurobiology. Certainly some would argue that the application of techniques and the experiential learning of what works and what doesn't is the path to take. But is this the best approach, in light of the knowledge that is now available to us? Does a medical doctor familiarize him or herself with only the symptoms and not the cause and mechanisms of an illness?

There is, I believe, much to be gained by understanding at least the fundamentals of brain function that play a critical role in our mental well-being. Freud, some will be surprised to learn, began his career as a neurobiologist, studying the nerves of crayfish with a view to forming an objective science of mental states based on neuroscientific research. Later he altered direction into psychoanalysis—research was not paying the bills, and the neuroscience of the day avoided the difficult subject of subjective experience and focused on the "nuts and bolts" of brain function. Now, with a greater understanding of both the subjective experience of the mind and the objective activities of the brain, the two disciplines of psychoanalysis and neuroscience can not only inform one another but integrate to provide a more mature and holistic understanding of mental well-being. The International Neuropsychoanalysis Society and our own efforts at The Neuropsychotherapist are just two examples of this attempt to integrate the best of both subjective and objective knowledge in mental health.

Consider the case of anxiety. If a therapist understood that chronic cortisol release due to anxiety can damage negative feedback loops that would normally attenuate the stress response (because excessive amounts of glucocorticoids damage activated glutamate synapses and pyramidal cells in the hippocampus and destabilize previously formed neural connections and neural/mental function in the hippocampus—see p, 25), he or she would not only have greater empathy for the struggling client, who finds it so difficult to relax or suffers from flashbacks or nightmares, but would also know that cognitive techniques are likely to prove ineffective until the underlying mechanisms are dealt with. The neurobiologically informed therapist would know that a "bottom up" approach, involving techniques that may be more physiological than psychological, is imperative to down-regulate a runaway stress response before cognitive approaches can have the desired effect.

Neuroscience can be a complicated subject, with its own academic terminology, often out of the grasp of the working therapist whose professional time is divided between clients, paperwork, and continuing education in his or her own niche of practice. There is often little time or desire to attempt to decipher the latest research from the *Journal of Neuroscience*—as I write this preface I note that the latest article in this journal is entitled "Densin-180 Controls the Trafficking and Signalling of L-Type Voltage-Gated $Ca_v1.2$ Ca^{2+} Channels at Excitatory Synapses", a subject that probably wouldn't get many psychotherapists motivated to give up a weekend to ponder how the discoveries of mice lacking densin could help their Monday-morning client with depression. This is where *The Neuropsychotherapist*, and this book, can help form a bridge between the world of neuroscience and the practical needs of the psychotherapist.

As an example, and not to dismiss the abovementioned article out of hand, there would be little point in my attempting to excite a counsellor about voltage-gated $Ca_v1.2$ channels playing a vital role in plasticity—that subject is too fine-grained, too full of mysterious jargon, and for the most part just plain tedious. But if I were to inform you there is a protein that helps signalling in the brain and contributes to the regulation of cognition and mood, and that it is part of a bigger puzzle of the molecular mechanism for a number of psychopathologies, then you may be more interested. What if there are ways to protect or enhance this protein and its pathway that are easy for anyone to grasp? The fine-grained science may sound like foreign gibberish, but the practical application of such knowledge may be just what your client needs.

Because our brain is an organ, like any other organ in our body, it is dependent on blood flow, oxygenation, nutrients, and signalling from other parts of the body. So the brain should be studied in context—the context of the whole body—just as the study of the mind entails the context of others and the environment. For this reason we also consider the influences of diet, gut microbes, the activity of the heart, inflammation, physical pain, gene expression, and other modulators of central-nervous-system activity. Most psychotherapists are aware of the importance of social systems and their impact on mental well-being; on a physiological level, the brain also functions in a systems context.

Does this mean the psychotherapist needs to be an expert in every area of neurobiology in order to understand clients effectively? No, but in addition to enhancing your own perspective and practise, awareness of what may be influencing the mental health of a client *beyond* the psychodynamic will help you identify needs that can be best met by the input of other specialists. There may be pathology that has resulted from a head injury, so that a neuropsychologist or neurologist is required. There may be a problem with a deficiency or overabundance of vitamins, minerals, or other chemicals in the client's system that requires the attention of a naturopath or medical doctor. Having an idea of what is going on "under the hood" will give you an edge in identifying problem areas that are beyond your area of expertise and greatly improving outcomes for your client by pointing them in the right direction.

As an illustration, I remember learning about the different ways inflammation can cause depression: as the immune system activates an inflammatory response, it can deplete the body of the serotonin precursor tryptophan. Inflammation can also influence noradrenergic activity, stimulating the hypothalamic–pituitary–adrenal (HPA) axis. One client who approached me for help was depressed and also suffering from a number of severe allergies. Knowing that the inflammatory response to the allergens was likely disrupting her serotonin production and activating her stress response through the HPA axis, I referred her to a naturopath for testing and treatment. When she returned about a month later, her symptoms of inflammation were significantly reduced—along with her symptoms of depression. This reprieve gave us the opportunity to work on deep-seated emotional issues, unhampered by a brain in a state of emergency due to allergy-induced inflammation. The client had not made the connection between her allergies and depression, but the inflammatory response was clearly a major factor. She still had psychotherapy work to do, but my knowledge of her neurobiology gave me enough insight to direct her to the right help. Having her inflammation under control gave her the energy and motivation to continue with effective psychotherapy.

It is my hope that this book will open your mind and encourage you to take a more holistic perspective than ever before. As therapists we are privileged to live in a time when breakthroughs in the neurobiological sciences are both confirming and informing vital aspects of psychotherapeutic practice, breaking down traditional barriers and stimulating multidisciplinary approaches that will ultimately revolutionize how we think about mental health. For the sake of those we seek to help, may this book form one step along the way to acquiring the best tools and knowledge available in the quest for real change and lasting well-being.

INTRODUCTION

The Psychotherapist's Essential Guide to the Brain provides an overview of the essential parts and functions of the brain that every modern-day therapist should be familiar with. Written in accessible language and consolidating a large body of neuroscientific knowledge, this handy "beginner's guide" forms a practical and accessible introduction to brain science for psychotherapists. The current chapter lays the groundwork for a big-picture view of how the brain functions, providing essential reference points from which the reader may go on to develop an understanding of what is happening in the brains of clients, as well as in his or her own.

The contemporary psychotherapist has access to a more sophisticated model of mental health than ever before, yet key elements of that model entail an understanding of the neural functions that underpin behaviour, relationships, personality, and a sense of self and the surrounding world. This guide aims to bridge the gap between the often esoteric realm of neuroscience research and the pragmatic realities of psychotherapy with clients. The therapist with a practical grasp of the concepts, regions and functions of the nervous system will be rewarded with improved outcomes that reflect a more holistic and integrated understanding of clients.

Since Freud, the brain has been variously conceived in terms of an electrical system, a chemical system, and, more recently, a highly interconnected electrochemical network. In terms of convention, we are only now emerging from an outdated medical model that conceptualized the brain primarily as a chemical system that could be "fixed" by means of drug intervention, and coming to the realization that the brain is a malleable communication network where the patterns of connections within and between brain regions are as important as the chemicals that serve the impulses travelling these routes.

Understanding this communication network, which happens to be the most complex system we know, can enhance our practice of psychotherapy as we tune in to the intricacies of its various attributes. As a stand-out example, understanding the basic concept of a fast-reacting limbic system versus a slower prefrontal cortex can shed light on why cognitive therapies are often largely ineffective until more basic emotional issues have been addressed via a "bottom up" approach. Or, understanding that emotional memories can be "unhinged" from the hippocampal time/space marker for an event can furnish not only greater empathy for the PTSD sufferer but also ideas on how to reintegrate the traumatic memories from the past so that they stop intruding on the now. We can create better interventions when we know that memory is everything when it comes to brain function, and that memories can change, our neural networks can be altered, and even genetic expressions that support those neural networks can change.

And so, with a debt to modern neuroscience, we embark on this modest overview of the brain, trusting it will serve you well in your conceptualizations of clients and arouse your curiosity for further learning.

A connectogram of a healthy control subject.

Connectograms are graphical representations of connectomics, the field of study dedicated to mapping and interpreting all of the white-matter fibre connections in the human brain. These circular graphs based on diffusion MRI data utilize graph theory to demonstrate the white-matter connections and cortical characteristics for single structures, single subjects, or populations.

In this image: From outside to inside, the rings represent the cortical region, grey matter volume, surface area, cortical thickness, curvature, degree of connectivity, node strength, betweenness centrality, eccentricity, nodal efficiency, and eigenvector centrality. Between degree of connectivity and node strength, a blank ring has been added as a placeholder. This connectogram includes five additional nodal measures not included in the standard connectogram.   Image: Wikipedia.

THE DIVIDED BRAIN

Iain McGilchrist, in his noteworthy book *The Master and His Emissary: The Divided Brain and the Making of the Western World* (2009), describes the asymmetry of the brain and the very different natures of the left and right hemispheres. This horizontal understanding of the mental system, as opposed to the vertical triune perspective, gives us insight into the distinctly different yet complementary functions of the two hemispheres. In short, the right hemisphere handles broad attention (what we attend to comes first to us through the right hemisphere); is good at making connections so that we can appreciate the wholeness of dynamic structures and relationships that change over time; is attuned to emotion; and is empathic, intuitive, and moral. In contrast, the left hemisphere has narrow attention; is good at deconstructing things into parts; and has an appreciation for static, decontextualized, inanimate structures and abstractions. McGilchrist (2009) summarizes the "two worlds" of the hemispheres in this way:

> The brain has to attend to the world in two completely different ways, and in so doing to bring two different worlds into being. In the one [that of the right hemisphere], we experience—the live, complex, embodied world of individual, always unique beings, forever in flux, a net of interdependencies, forming and reforming wholes, a world with which we are deeply connected. In the other [that of the left hemisphere] we "experience" our experience in a special way: a "re-presented" version of it, containing now static, separable, bounded, but essentially fragmented entities, grouped into classes, on which predictions can be based. This kind of attention isolates, fixes and makes each thing explicit by bringing it under the spotlight of attention. In doing so it renders things inert, mechanical, lifeless. But it also enables us for the first time to know, and consequently to learn and to make things. This gives us power. (p. 31)

Allan Schore explains that the early-maturing right hemisphere is the locus of attachment formation and essentially the gateway to affect regulation later in life—so much so, indeed, that developing an expanded capacity for right-hemisphere processing (an emphasis on right-brained affective skills rather than a left–cognitive bias) is central to clinical expertise (Schore, 2012). In a similar vein, Badenoch (2008) warns therapists to be grounded in right-brain engagement with clients or run the risk of being disengaged from the regulating and integrating influence of right brain-to-right brain connection with clients. She further encourages therapists to widen their window of tolerance, be conscious of implicit vulnerabilities, and develop mindfulness to be present with both the client and self. There is a place for left-brain focus when thinking about specific interventions, but as McGilchrist admonishes, the left should remain servant to the right hemisphere as master.

Left Hemisphere

- Less white matter—prioritizing local information transfer within regions, reflected in an increased ability to localize attention and enhancing its self-referring nature.
- More reliant on dopamine.
- Superior in the expression of anger.
- Highly focused attention to detail; local, narrowly focused attention—sees "parts".
- Attends narrowly to the right field of view, the right side of the body, the right side of objects (demonstrated in what is known as "hemi-neglect" following a right-hemisphere stroke).
- More engaged with the known, the learned, the expected; prefers what it knows—"grasps" what is in focus and has been prioritized.
- Efficient when routine is predictable.
- Finds solutions perceived to fit best with current knowledge or schemas
- Processes information in an increasingly focal way that suppresses information not immediately relevant.
- Suppresses the right-hemisphere ability to make distant associations among words or objects (and the broader scope of attention in general).
- Takes a local, short-term view.
- Identifies things by labels rather than context; does not deduce from context like the right hemisphere—in conversation takes things more literally and has difficulty understanding implied meaning. Things are decontextualized and interpreted by an internal logic.
- Proficient at abstraction—storing and manipulating information in abstracted types, classes, categories, and representations that are impersonal, fixed, and equivalent. Recognizes objects in a category in a generic, non-specific way, but not the uniqueness of individuals.
- Codes non-living things and has an affinity for the mechanical.
- Better at identifying simple shapes that are easily categorized.
- Interested in the utility of things—machines, tools, man-made things.
- Sees one's own body as an assemblage of parts from which it maintains a level of detachment.
- More sophisticated in language and symbol manipulation, with greater vocabulary and more subtle and complex syntax than the right hemisphere.

Right Hemisphere

- More white matter—facilitating faster transfer of information across regions, reflected in an increased ability to hold global attention.
- More sensitive to testosterone.
- More reliant on noradrenaline.
- More intimately connected with the limbic system—identifies emotions faster and more accurately than the left and is more involved in emotional expression (except anger).
- Open to broad awareness; on the lookout in a broad and flexible way with vigilance and global sustained attention—sees the "whole".
- Processes information in a non-focal manner.
- Attends to the peripheral field of vision and the entire left–right visual field.
- Alert and attentive to the new and the novel—awareness begins in the right hemisphere, grounding and integrating the experience, before being further processed in the left on a more detailed level.
- More engaged in the learning of new information—explores.
- Outperforms the left when prediction is difficult; more capable of shifting the frame of reference (important for problem solving).
- Can associate words or objects that are not closely related; can understand unfamiliar (non-cliché) metaphor.
- Better able to integrate perceptual processes from different senses.
- Longer working memory.
- Recognizes broad or complex patterns.
- More involved in insight and deductive reasoning.
- Sees things in context and in terms of relationships; attentive to context in conversation—vital for a sense of humour.
- Can recognize the individual and uniqueness within a category, such as recognizing individual faces in the category of faces.
- Interested in the personal, the living, rather than the impersonal and non-living.
- Plays a primary role in empathy, the theory of "mind", identification with others, social interaction, and emotional understanding.
- Connected with the self as an embodied whole.
- Specializes in non-verbal communication, the implicit, subtle unconscious perceptions, emotional shifts, subtle clues and meanings.
- Gives an appreciation of depth in time and space.

THREE LAYERS

A well-known model of the human brain is that described by neuroscientist Paul MacLean as the triune brain (MacLean, 1990). This evolutionary view of the brain describes three main regions in an evolutionary hierarchy: the primitive "reptilian" complex (the brainstem), the "palaeomammalian" complex (the limbic system), and the "neomammalian" complex (the cortex). The reptilian complex is fully developed at birth, while the palaeomammalian complex is partly developed and continues to develop during early childhood, and the neomammalian complex is mostly underdeveloped at birth and is the last part of the triune brain to develop (The Neuropsychotherapy Institute, 2014c). The implications of the model are that the survival instincts of the palaeomammalian complex (the limbic system) are significantly developed during the early years of life, distinct from the later-developing cognitive processes of the neomammalian complex (Rossouw, 2011). More sophisticated contemporary models of the brain and behaviour do not fully support MacLean's evolutionary model (the brain is much more integrated and seamless than MacLean's model might suggest); however, the "bottom-up" perspective of development remains instructive for a corresponding bottom-up therapeutic approach (Rossouw, 2011). This bottom-up approach, as distinct from a top-down, cognitive approach, looks to establish safety through down-regulation of sympathetic over-arousal and activation of a state of parasympathetic security, resulting in increased cortical blood flow to the left frontal cortex for effective activation of cognitive abilities, and limiting "looping" activity within the limbic system (Rossouw, 2011, p. 4) to allow for effective new learning.

The Primitive Brain (Reptilian Complex)

This system of the brain is responsible for the most basic survival functions, such as heart rate, breathing, body temperature, and orientation in space. Needless to say, functions like heart rate and breathing are of considerable importance, and the control mechanisms in this part of the brain are accordingly consistent.

It is important to recognize that the functions of the primitive brain will take precedence over other brain activity. For example, if you try to hold your breath (a prefrontal cortex-initiated activity), you will find that as carbon dioxide builds up in your bloodstream, this primitive part of your brain is going to want to take over and make you breathe again. Through training you may be able to increase your resistance to the basic urge to breathe, but inevitably you will eventually give in and take a breath.

Such threats to survival are first addressed by the primitive brain—as illustrated in "peripheral shutdown", where blood vessels on the periphery of the body are constricted in anticipation of physical trauma—and are prioritized over less vital functions.

The Limbic System (Paleomammalian Complex)

Sometimes referred to as the "emotional brain", the limbic system is the reactive part of us that initiates the "fight or flight" response to danger. Key areas of interest to psychotherapy are the hippocampus, the amygdala, and the hypothalamus. These form a very fast subconscious evaluation and response system designed to keep us safe.

The amygdala is like an early-warning system, with the motto "safety first"—put that safety plan into effect before consulting the executive brain (the new cortex). Picture yourself jumping out of the way of a snake-like object before closer examination reveals it to be just a garden hose in the grass. This is a very important first response, because if it were left to the prefrontal cortex to initiate, for example, a leap out of the way of a bus you had inadvertently stepped in front of, then it might be too late: that evaluation system is too slow. The amygdala makes very fast, albeit not always accurate, evaluations and has a fast track from the thalamus (incoming information) through to the hypothalamus that can initiate a stress response to forestall impending doom. The hippocampus plays an equally important role by encoding events in time and space and consolidating them from short-term to long-term memory.

Of particular interest to therapists is the case where the limbic system gets the cues wrong: where there is no danger in actuality, but the body is thrown into stress response anyway. From chronic low-grade stress to full-blown panic attacks, a maladaptive limbic system could be the key to what is troubling your client.

The New Cortex (Neomammalian Complex)

The new cortex is our "smart" brain, the executive part of our system that is responsible for all higher-order conscious activity such as language, abstract thought, imagination, and creativity, to name just a few. It also houses much of our memory—not just our biographical memory, but all of the automatic memories essential to talking, writing, walking, playing the piano, and countless other familiar activities (keep in mind, however, that the division of the brain into three large parts is a highly simplified conception: functionally the connectivity between all these regions greatly blurs the boundaries).

Of special interest to therapists is the prefrontal cortex—the part of the brain right behind our forehead—which may be slower in responding to incoming information than the limbic system, but is much more sophisticated in its processing. Such "slow" thinking is the hallmark of our human intelligence. Complex and new thinking on technical, emotional, social, and logical planes takes place here. It is where we can be rational and logical, creative and inventive. But, significantly, the prefrontal cortex can be "hijacked" by the limbic system in the event of a perceived threat (whether imagined or real). Our prefrontal can "go offline" as blood flow is directed to the deeper limbic system, the first responder in a priority one mission to keep us safe.

AMAZINGLY NETWORKED

The human brain has about 100,000 miles of white matter (bundles of myelinated axons) shooting electrochemical signals down 100 billion neurons through 100 trillion synaptic connections1—we are spectacularly connected!

The pattern of neural connectivity in our brains has long captured the attention of neuroanatomists. It can be described at several levels of scale: the individual synaptic connections that link individual neurons, networks connecting neuronal populations, and entire brain regions linked by white-matter highways. Mapping the large-scale connectivity within and between brain regions is what has captured the imagination of the National Institutes of Health in the US, which has funded the Human Connectome Project (HCP), a $40 million effort to map the human brain. Each of us has a unique neural map, rather like the uniqueness of our fingerprints, that has been shaped by our genetics, environment, and life experiences. It is this map, or "connectome", that researchers would like to recreate in a virtual space to model the highways and byways of neural connectivity.

The connectome is extremely complex and not yet well understood. It is the hope of the HCP that by mapping many individuals, they will establish a baseline of normal connectivity and reveal how connectivity differs across individuals displaying psychopathology.

In a recent study published in Nature Neuroscience (Smith et al., 2015), investigators found a significant relationship between the brain's default-mode network and personal traits such as IQ, language skills, and life satisfaction. The researchers examined 461 subjects, looking at the correlations between their resting-state functional connectivity and behavioural and demographic measures. They found that the subjects who returned high scores for cognition, memory, education, and income level—as opposed to more "negative" measures such as substance use and aggression—showed higher connectivity in components of their default network. Such connections included the medial frontal and parietal cortex, the temporo-parietal junction, the anterior insula, and the frontal operculum. This correlation between attributes of positive life functionality and underlying brain connectivity was interesting indeed—but did higher connectivity between components of the default network give rise to more "positive" life outcomes, or were there other developmental, relational, and environmental factors at play? The researchers admit that it was impossible to tell from their study. However, as causal relationships are progressively better

White matter fibre architecture from the Connectome Scanner dataset. The fibres are colour-coded by direction: red = left–right, green = anterior–posterior, blue = ascending–descending (RGB = XYZ).
Courtesy of the Laboratory of Neuro Imaging and the Athinoula A. Martinos Center for Biomedical Imaging, Consortium of the Human Connectome Project. www.humanconnectomeproject.org

understood, it may become feasible to use this information to assist a transition in the brain toward the positive axis.

Interestingly, one of the factors that most impacted the brain toward the negative axis was marijuana use

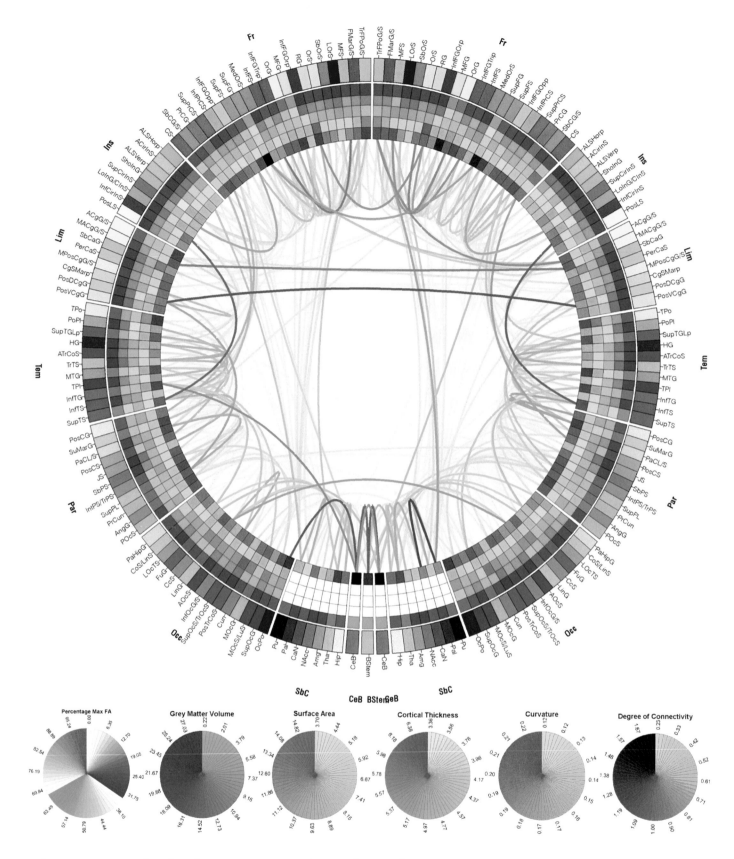

A connectogram showing the average connections and cortical measures of 110 normal, right-handed males, aged 25–36. Image by John Darrell Van Horn—PLoS One: http://journals.plos.org/plosone/article?id=10.1371/journal.pone.0037454

Van Horn, J. D., Irimia, A., Torgerson, C. M., Chambers, M. C., Kikinis, R., & Toga, A. W. (2012). Mapping connectivity damage in the case of Phineas Gage. PLoS ONE, 7(5):e37454. doi:10.1371/journal.pone.0037454 within the few weeks prior to the study. Such findings should raise a red flag and highlight the importance of more research to determine how marijuana affects the brain.

In addition to mapping the adult brain, the HCP has a developmental arm based at King's College London, Imperial College London, and Oxford University. It is the Developing Human Connectome Project (dHCP), whose aim is to break new ground with the creation of four-dimensional connectomes of early life. The project is looking to map brain connectivity from 20 to 44 weeks that will link clinical, behavioural, and genetic information to the connectome image.

Massive change occurs in the developing brain of a child, and the challenge to map and understand it is substantial. One of the studies the dHCP is currently engaged in involves 8-year-old children, half of whom were born prematurely and half full-term, to see if there are any brain network differences between them. Premature babies are at greater risk of neuro-developmental problems, but little is known about how they develop such impairments. A huge amount of brain development in infants occurs just prior to full term, and for that development to take place outside the mother, in the case of pre-terms, may be significant for these children. For instance, the fibres forming connections to and from the thalamus, the central exchange centre of the brain, grow extensively during the time period in which dHCP teams monitor premature babies. A map of this area during these critical developmental stages could yield valuable insights.

One of the principal investigators, David Edwards, says that there are structures being developed in the last trimester that may underlie conditions like schizophrenia, autism, and depression, and it is his hope that the project can identify subtle differences in connectivity that may predispose some children to mental illness.

A recent study at the University of California, San Francisco (Chang et al., 2016) demonstrated measurable differences in the connective wiring of children with sensory processing disorder (SPD) compared to typically developing children. The study is the largest ever conducted with child SPD sufferers and the first to compare white-matter tracts in the brains of typically developing children against those with SPD.

The imaging done with these children detected abnormalities in the SPD subjects in the white-matter tracts that serve as connections for the auditory, visual, and somatosensory (tactile) systems involved in sensory processing, including in the connections between left and right hemispheres. The abnormal microstructure of sensory white matter tracts in children with SPD likely alters the timing of sensory transmission, so that the processing of sensory stimuli and the integration of information across multiple senses becomes difficult or impossible.

The imaging results showed a stronger correlation with the direct measurements of tactile and auditory processing taken during the neurological testing than with the parent report survey, which the researchers put down to the likelihood that the direct measurements were more objective.

Another impressive tool employed by researchers mapping the connectome is the connectogram, a two-dimensional graph used to study the arrangement of white-matter fibre in the brain. Based on diffusion MRI data, this circular graph highlights the strength of connections between different regions of the brain. The connectogram can display 83 cortical regions within each hemisphere, and unlike other representations of the connectome that require software to display the three dimensions, these representations can show connected regions in a flat, two-dimensional graph.

The left half of the connectogram depicts the left hemisphere, and the right half depicts the right hemisphere. The circular graph is further broken down into sections representing the frontal lobe, insular cortex, limbic lobe, temporal lobe, parietal lobe, occipital lobe, subcortical structures, and cerebellum. The brain stem is also represented, between the two hemispheres at the bottom of the graph. Each cortical area within the lobes is labelled and features a unique colour that can be used to designate the same cortical region in other figures, so that the reader can find the corresponding cortical area on a geometrically accurate surface and see exactly how disparate the connected regions may be. Inside the cortical surface ring are concentric circles representing different attributes of the corresponding cortical regions. In order from outermost to innermost, these metric rings represent the grey matter volume, surface area, cortical thickness, curvature, and degree of connectivity. The lines in the diagram on the facing page show the connections between regions. The opacity and colour of the lines represent the strength of the connection.

Our brains are wonderfully and complexly connected, and the cutting-edge research currently revealing the connectome is leading us to highly objective assessment using quantifiable biomarkers. This will not only yield a more refined and sophisticated definition of pathology, but may lead to much more personalized treatments in the days to come.

NEURONS

Our genes provide an organizational map for the development of our brains. While some designation of the place and function of neurons is fixed by coding genes, other functional aspects are subject to the influence of experience, in the form of non-coding genes that make up the so-called "nurture" part of our genetic expression (The Neuropsychotherapy Institute, 2014a). Our genetic blueprint, along with epigenetic (experience dependent) expression of genes and memory formation, creates a complex neural communication system throughout the nervous system, which is itself a complexity of synaptic/dendritic connections modulated by neurochemicals.

The nervous system has two main divisions of cells: nerve cells (neurons), and glial cells (glia). Glial cells have traditionally been recognized as a kind of support network for neurons, providing many essential functions to facilitate the neural network. However, they have more recently been acknowledged to form a communication network themselves, working in tandem with neurons (Keleman, 2013; Verkhratsky & Butt, 2007). The function of a neuron is determined by where it is in the brain, how it is connected with neighbouring cells, and its individual functional character. Take the analogy of a human individual: our function in society is determined by where we are, who we are connected to, and how we interact with others and our environment (Cozolino, 2014). The anatomist János Szentágothai estimated that our individual neurons are able to contact any other neuron via no more than six interneuronal connections (Drachman, 2005). This "six degrees of separation" has become a popular social idea—that people are connected six or fewer steps from each other in a "friend of a friend" relationship—popularized by the play and film Six Degrees of Separation by John Guare in the early 1990s and followed by numerous books, films, and TV shows based on the same idea.

While there are different types of nerve cells performing a variety of functions, it is helpful to consider a generic model that represents the fundamentals of all neurons. The figure to the left illustrates the main components of the neuron (see Chapter 2 of Kandel, Schwartz, Jessell, Siegelbaum, & Hudspeth, 2012, for a comprehensive description of neuron physiology).

Neurons communicate by means of two primary processes that have been comprehensively studied: an electrical signal within the neuron, and chemical signals between neurons. Using various chemicals known as neurotransmitters, neurons transmit signals across a very small gap between cells in an area known as the synaptic cleft. Most neurons can send and receive signals by different types of neurotransmitters, and different neurotransmitters work at different speeds (The Neuropsychotherapy Institute, 2014a).

DENDRITES

CELL BODY

NUCLEUS

DIRECTION OF NERVE IMPULSE

MYELIN SHEATH

AXON

AXON TERMINALS

SYNAPSE

The figure below is a radically simplified representation of a synapse. The upper part represents the presynaptic terminal of one cell's axon, and the lower part the postsynaptic dendrite of another cell. Communication flows from the presynaptic terminal to the dendrites of a neighbouring cell. Dendrites are like the branches of a tree that spread out to reach other cells, and are the main areas for receiving incoming signals (Kandel et al., 2012).

Synaptic vesicles are packets of neurotransmitters that migrate to special release sites called active zones. These packets come to the surface of the presynaptic terminal and release their contents, by a process known as exocytosis, into the synaptic cleft. The released molecules diffuse across the gap, and some are received by receptors on the opposite-facing dendrite. The receptor sites on the dendrite bind to specific neurotransmitters, producing either an inhibiting or excitatory effect on the receiving cell. This occurs via an opening of ion channels in the membrane of the cell that essentially produces a membrane potential in the dendrite (a positive or negative charge within the cell). There can be many different types of ions in neurons, but the most common are sodium ions (Na+) and potassium ions (K+), and it is the balance of Na+ and K+ inside and outside the cell that determines the overall "charge" or potential of the cell. This balance is regulated by sodium–potassium pumps that continually exchange Na+ inside the cell for K+ outside the cell. The more positively charged a neuron becomes, the more likely it will pass a certain threshold of potential (e.g., from −70 mV to −67 mV), in a process called depolarization, and "fire". Conversely, an increase in the membrane potential (e.g., from −70 mV to −72 mV), known as hyperpolarization, decreases the likelihood of the neuron firing. Depolarizations are termed excitatory postsynaptic potentials (EPSPs) because they increase the likelihood of firing, and hyperpolarizations are termed inhibitory postsynaptic potentials (IPSPs) because they have the opposite effect. Neurons have a resting potential somewhere between −60 and −70 mV, whereas glia cells measure between −80 and −90 mV (Lewis et al., 2011).

Ionotropic receptors, such as AMPA, accept transmitters that directly alter the receiving cell's potential, and are thus fast-acting, whereas NMDA receptors require prior activation of the postsynaptic neuron through another channel before its ion channel can be opened (see Grawe, 2007, pp. 36–37). Some neurotransmitters will cause the receiving dendrite to become more positively charged, and others will cause the dendrite to become more negatively charged. The receiving dendrite "sums" the incoming chemical signals to arrive at a resultant synaptic potential which is then communicated to the main body of the cell. All of these signals are summed at the beginning of the axon, at the axon initial segment (Bender & Trussell, 2012). If the resulting charge rises above a resting potential, an electrical signal flows down the axon to the presynaptic terminals, causing the membrane of each terminal to open up channels allowing calcium into the cell. In turn, this causes the synaptic vesicles to release their chemicals into the synaptic cleft.

2 NERVE IMPULSE

PRESYNAPTIC NEURON

MITOCHONDRION

1 NEUROTRANSMITTERS ARE SYNTHESIZED AND STORED INTO THE VESICLES

VOLATGE GATED Ca^{2+} CHANNEL

NEUROTRANSMITTER RE-UPTAKE

4 NEUROTRANSMITTERS RELEASED INTO THE SYNAPTIC SPACE VIA EXOCYTOSIS

5 NEUROTRANSMITTER BINDS TO THE RECEPTOR MOLECULES AND OPENS LIGAND-GATED ION CHANNEL

Ca^{2+}

3 DEPOLARIZATION CAUSES VOLTAGE GATED Ca^{2+} CHANNEL OPENING AND Ca^{2+} ENTERS INTO THE AXON TERMINAL

AXON TERMINAL

SYNAPTIC SPACE

POSTSYNAPTIC MEMBRANE

LIGAND-GATED ION CHANNEL

POSTSYNAPTIC NEURON

This (albeit simplified) description of the process illustrates the binary nature of neurotransmitters in either initiating an action potential or not.

The figure on the previous page also shows some of the neurotransmitters being reabsorbed into the presynaptic terminal. Such uptake, via plasma membrane transporters, serves two purposes: recapturing the chemicals for reuse, and terminating the synaptic action of the cell (Kandel et al., 2012). Drugs used to inhibit the re-uptake of neurotransmitters will, in effect, keep the neurotransmitter in the vicinity of the postsynaptic dendrite, so that when receptors are available for that particular chemical, they will bind with it. Thus, antidepressants are designed to inhibit serotonin re-uptake, keeping it in the synaptic cleft and prolonging postsynaptic activation (The Neuropsychotherapy Institute, 2014b). Another process whereby neurotransmitters are removed from the synaptic cleft is degradation, in which enzymes chemically break down the neurotransmitter and the resulting molecules are taken up by the presynaptic terminal. Within the presynaptic terminal, the neurotransmitter is then reassembled and repackaged for release once again. Finally, glial cells also remove neurotransmitters from the synaptic space to prevent further interaction with the postsynaptic cell.

Activation Patterns

A single neuron does not produce much information on its own through firing or not firing. Firing entails a certain rate, intensity, and resulting neurotransmitter output at the synapse. A single neuron simply responds to specific inputs from other neurons, or directly from the environment in the case of sensory cells. To make sense of the flow of information coming from our sensory organs, the neural system is organized into a hierarchy of increasingly complex networks. One hundred billion individual neurons, boasting and average of 7,000–10,000 synaptic connections each, together contribute to neural network profiles that represent an aspect of brain function (such as perceiving a particular sound), and these profiles integrate with many others to form various functions of our nervous system, some of which are concentrated in different areas of the brain (Siegel, 2012).

The hierarchy of neural networks is organized from sensory input to the perception of complex objects/understandings to even more complex cognitive and affective processes. For example, the "raw" visual data streamed from the sensory input of the retina is recognized by neurons in a fragmented fashion whereby individual parts of the scene are processed by neurons tuned to "recognize" small, specific elements. These fragments are then assembled by more complex neural networks involving higher-order cells that recognize the assembly of the parts. At the top of the hierarchy are cells and networks in the cortex that recognize the "whole picture". Once this broader perception is realized, further cognitive/affective processes can occur as a result of this input. The flow of information is not serial but a complexity of parallel processing that utilizes feedback from various brain regions. There is no neuron that can recognize the complexities of an object like a chair. Only through the summation of complex networks, and with experience, can we recognize a chair for what it is. Nor is there a single area of the brain that handles a specific mental function in isolation. Just as neurons do not perceive on their own, neural profiles activate and integrate with other regions across the nervous system (Siegel, 2012).

The brain is further organized into functional systems that to some extent can be identified by elements of the physical architecture of the central nervous system. From a single sensory input neuron, the scale of operations increases to complex hierarchies of neural networks that form maps representing input features in specific areas of the cortex. These complex signals are in turn processed within broad functional systems of organization according to the physical architecture of the brain. Such functional architecture is currently being mapped by the Human Connectome Project (http://www.humanconnectomeproject.org).

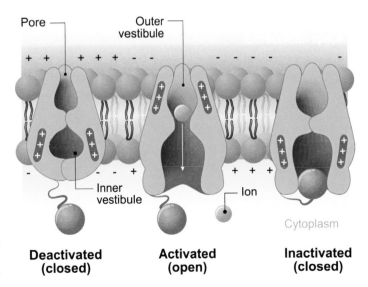

Above: Voltage-gated channels found along the axon and synapse of neurons propagate electrical signals down the neuron

GLIA THE OVERLOOKED CELLS

The brain contains two major classes of cells: neurons and glia. While both are neural cells, conventionally, the fundamental difference between the two classes has been understood to be that neurons are electrically excitable, whereas glia are non-excitable. Various types of glial cells make up about 90% of all cells in the human brain. In the central nervous system, they are referred to as macroglial or neuroglial cells, and can be categorized into three types: astrocytes, oligodendrocytes, and ependymal cells (Verkhratsky & Butt, 2007).

Glial cells have traditionally been regarded as passive supporting cells. The name *glia* is from Greek, literally meaning "glue". Rudolf Ludwig Karl Virchow (1821–1902), who coined the term for neuroscience, thought of glia as a sort of "nerve putty"—a connective tissue void of any cellular elements (Verkhratsky & Butt, 2007). However, today we have a very different understanding of the function of glia in the nervous system. Glia play a vital role in the growth and development of neurons as well as their maintenance and death. Atroglial cells provide the stem elements to birth neurons; they compartmentalize neurons, synapses, and capillaries into functional units and help modulate chemical signals between neurons. Oligodendroglia even myelinate the axons of neurons in the central nervous system (as Schwann cells do in the peripheral nervous system), creating faster communication pathways.

In 1984, researchers discovered that astrocytes and oligodendrocytes possessed GABA receptors. GABA (*Gamma-aminobutyric acid*) is an inhibitory neurotransmitter that plays a counterpart role to the glutamates, if glutamate is the accelerator of the brain, GABA is the brake. A few years later, others found that astroglial cells can communicate over long distances by propagating calcium waves. Since then it has been demonstrated that glial cells can express practically every type of neurotransmitter and can detect the activity of neighbouring neurons. In fact, far from being mere passive, non-excitable glue for neurons, glia form a whole other communication circuit in tandem with the neuronal circuit, the two systems communicating with each other via chemical and electrical signalling.

The communication network of glia is what Stanley Keleman (2013) has called the "slow brain"—a support system for a wide order of connections and cortical growth. This slower system is vitally connected to the voluntary muscular signalling from the body which has a bidirectional effect on the brain and body posture and responses.

Much is still being discovered about these cells that make up the greater part of our brain, but what is not in doubt is that there is much more to glia than we ever imagined.

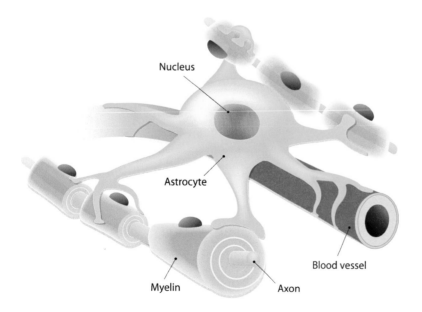

Astrocytes (meaning "star-like cells") are the most abundant cells in the central nervous system. This simplistic diagram shows an astrocyte forming the scaffolding for a number of neuron axons and a blood vessel. The blue myelin around the axons originates from oligodendrocytes (not shown here).

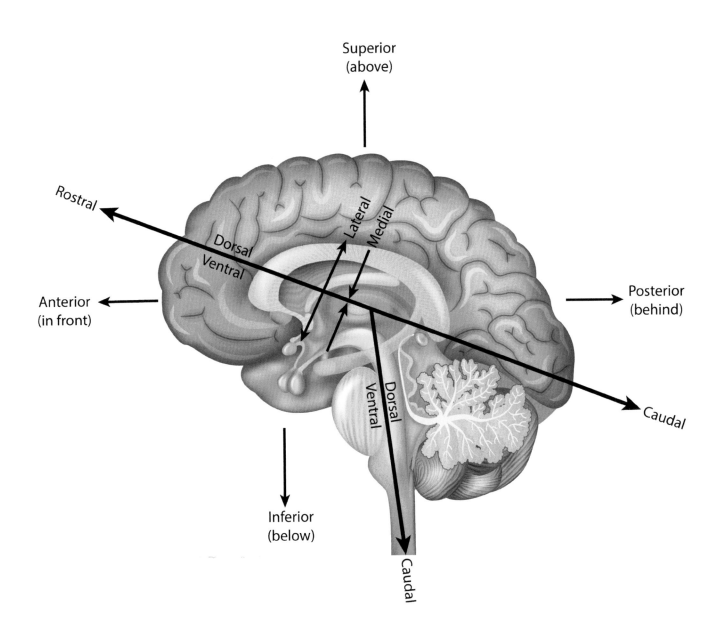

Location Terminology	
Anterior	relating to the front or to the nose end
Dorsal	relating to the back or toward the surface of the back or top of the head
Lateral	relating to the sides or away from the midline
Ventral	relating to the underside or toward the surface of the chest or bottom of the head
Parietal	relating to the wall of the body or of a body cavity or hollow structure
Medial	relating to the middle or the midline
Basal	relating to the bottom layer or base

Planes	
Horizontal	Horizontal sections are the images of the brain you would see as if from directly above or from directly below (the dorsal or ventral perspective)
Sagittal	The sagittal sections are the side-on views, like the image above
Frontal	The frontal sections are views from the anterior or posterior perspective
Cross	The cross sections are views from a rostral/caudal perspective

DEEP SYSTEMS

THE LIMBIC SYSTEM

The limbic system (also known as the paleomammalian brain) is a collection of brain structures located in the middle of the brain. It was first defined by Paul Broca in the 19th century as the structures between the cerebral hemisphere and the brainstem (i.e., the limbus, or border of the brain). The limbic system is not a discrete system itself but rather a collection of structures—anatomically related but varying greatly in function. The term has been in use for about 70 years, despite the belief of some neuroscientists that it should be abandoned for implying that the various structures represent a functionally unified system. Irrespective of terminology, collectively we can think of the limbic system as the centre for emotional responsiveness, motivation, memory formation and integration, olfaction, and the mechanisms designed to keep us safe. These are broad strokes, certainly—not to suggest that the neocortex is not involved in these functions, but these are the focal activities of the limbic system. For the purposes of this overview we will be considering the amygdala, hippocampus, and hypothalamus as the main limbic structures of clinical relevance to the practising psychotherapist. We will also touch on the thalamus, which feeds the limbic system with sensory input.

The basal ganglia, a set of subcortical structures located near the thalamus and hypothalamus, are also included in the limbic system and are involved in intentional movements. The limbic system is closely connected to the prefrontal cortex, and it is this prefrontal–limbic connection that is strengthened when practising mindfulness. The functional relevance of the limbic system to psychotherapy is obvious, as affect, memory, sensory processing, time perception, attention, consciousness, autonomic control, motor behaviour, and more are all mediated in and through this collection of structures.

AC Anterior commissure
AN Anterior nucleus of thalamus
DG Dentate gyrus
FR Fasciculus retroflexus
IN Interpeduncular nucleus
LT Lamina terminalis
MB Mammillary body
MD Mediodorsal thalamic nucleus
MF Medial forebrain bundle
MT Mammillothalmic tract
NA Nucleus accumbens
OB Olfactory bulbs
OC Optic chiasm
OL Olfactory striae lateral
OS Olfactory striae medial
OT Olfactory tract
PG Pituitary gland
PT Paraterminal gyrus
SA Subcallosal area
SM Stria medullaris
SN Septal nuclei
SP Septum pellucidum
ST Stria terminallis

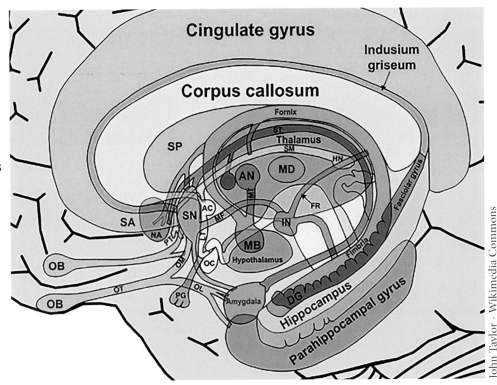

John Taylor - Wikimedia Commons

This diagram shows some of the complexity of the limbic system. Note how the olfactory bulbs feed directly into the amygdala, giving smell a particularly important role in emotional memory and evaluation of circumstances—we can smell danger faster than our "smart brain" will recognize a problem, and we can automatically recall the emotions of a past love at the smell of the perfume they used to wear. It is also striking that the size of these structures has little correlation to their power and importance in this amazing system.

THE THALAMUS

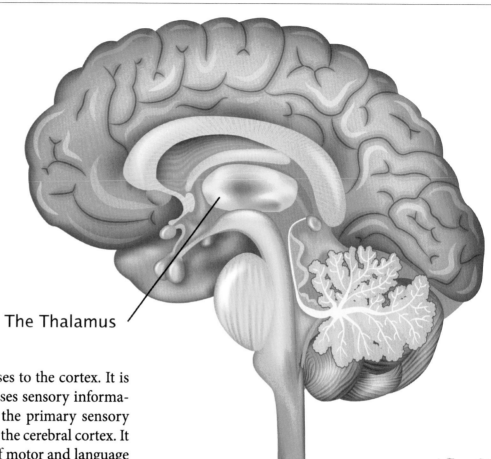

The thalamus (from the Greek word meaning "chamber") is centrally located between the cerebral cortex and the midbrain and is known for its role in relaying sensory and motor signals to the cerebral cortex, and in the regulation of sleep, consciousness, and alertness—rather like a hub

The Thalamus

of information flow from the senses to the cortex. It is believed that the thalamus processes sensory information in addition to relaying it to the primary sensory areas and receiving feedback from the cerebral cortex. It plays major roles in the support of motor and language systems and (in connection with the hippocampus) the spatial memory that is critical for episodic memory.

Interestingly, a common genetic variation in humans is that of the serotonin transporter 5-HTTLPR. People who inherit two short alleles (SERT-ss) also have more neurons and larger volume in parts of the thalamus. The SERT-ss inheritance is linked to a greater vulnerability to depression, PTSD, and suicide. The dorsal thalamus also plays a role in the inhibition of compulsive behaviour—we will examine this more closely later, when we consider the so-called OCD loop that involves the orbitofrontal cortex, striatum, and thalamus.

The thalamus is important for sleep regulation, in particular slow-wave sleep cycles, and coordinates parts of the cortex as sleep changes from state to state—the latter in orchestration with the activity of the hippocampus.

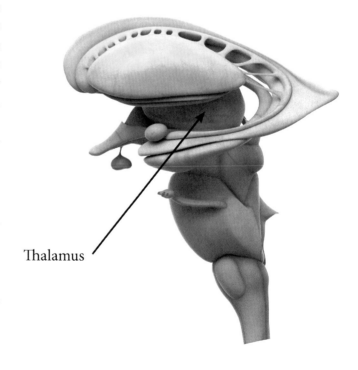

Thalamus

In sum, the thalamus appears to play a greater role than merely the relay of sensory information and is integral to brain function in a cortico–thalamo–cortical pathway of processing.

THE AMYGDALA

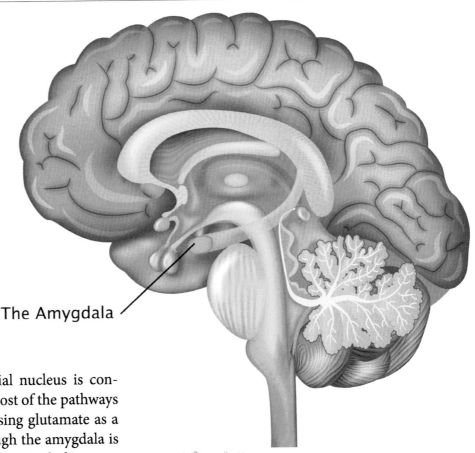

The amygdala is located in both hemispheres of the brain and is involved in a range of cognitive processes. The lateral amygdala receives input from visual, auditory, and somatosensory systems: the central nucleus is connected with the brainstem that controls innate behaviour and associated physiological responses, while the medial nucleus is connected with the olfactory system. Most of the pathways into the amygdala are excitatory, using glutamate as a transmitter. Information flow through the amygdala is modulated by a number of transmitters, including norepinephrine, serotonin, dopamine, and acetylcholine.

The amygdala forms part of the limbic system. It is most commonly recognized as the emotional processing centre that receives incoming sensory information and processes it for an emotional response. The response may be a defence to a perceived threat, a critical function of this "early-warning system". The amygdala learns how to respond to various stimuli based on its reference to implicit memory and makes decisions on how to initiate an emotional reaction to such stimuli. The emotional memory learned and utilized by the amygdala is episodic–autobiographical memory that can be notably implicit or unconscious, in contrast with explicit or declarative memory processed by the hippocampus.

The left and right amygdalae have separate memory systems, but they work together to evaluate incoming information and process an emotional response, encoding, storing and retrieving memories that are associated with certain cues in the environment. The right amygdala is more strongly associated with nega-

The Amygdala

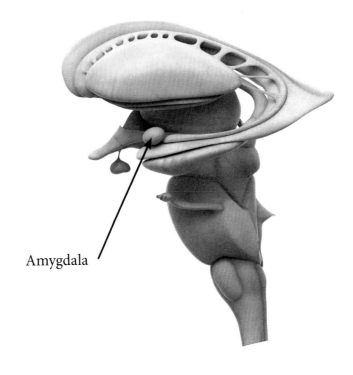

Amygdala

tive emotions such as fear and sadness, whereas the left amygdala has been associated with both positive and negative emotional responses.

The amygdala has an attentional role, focusing our attention on the most important stimuli in the environment. It helps us define a stimulus and primes our immediate response, for example in recognizing a dangerous stimulus and initiating a stress response. Processing social cues (e.g., evaluating faces) is also part of what the amygdala does prior to these cues being processed in higher cortical areas like the medial prefrontal cortex. Evaluating faces (e.g., the trustworthiness of a face) is an important social processing skill that is carried out very quickly in the limbic system. The amygdala also plays a part in processing reward learning and the resulting motivation, and modulating emotional states such as aggression, maternal instincts, and sexual and digestion behaviours as well as attention, perception, and explicit memory—generally thought to be part of processing the emotional significance of what we are encountering. Such processing causes the amygdala to respond with the release of hormones, or neuromodulators, that can alter the cognitive processing in cortical areas as well as activate the body for an appropriate response via the hypothalamus.

In terms of information flow, sensory input goes to the thalamus and then directly to the amygdala (except olfaction, which goes directly to the amygdala), while it is sent also via a slower path to the neocortex. The amygdala is especially activated by surprising, ambiguous, and uncertain situations or stimuli. If the amygdala perceives a correspondence between the record of experiences in the hippocampus and incoming information, and judges that the stimulus warrants a fight, flight, or freeze response, then it will trigger the hypothalamic–pituitary–adrenal (HPA) axis and "hijack" the prefrontal cortex (PFC), partly in the form of blood flow being redirected from the PFC to the limbic system. This amygdala activity processes information milliseconds earlier than the neocortex, so in the case where implicit memory matches an incoming stimulus, the amygdala acts before any possible direction from the neocortex can be received. On the other hand, if the amygdala does not perceive a match to the incoming stimulus, it acts according to the directions received from the neocortex. This means that when the amygdala perceives a threat, it initiates a response to keep us safe from that threat, although this may not be the most adaptive response. We know a lot more about the fear response of the amygdala than its other functions, but there is likely much more going on in this structure than we yet realize.

In the case of depression, the amygdala is often found to be enlarged from continual hyperactivation, with studies showing that there is an increased metabolic activity in the amygdala of depressed subjects. There is a positive correlation between the degree of amygdala activation and the severity of the depression. The depressive symptoms do not seem to dampen the anxiety-readiness for negative events or the ability to recall negative memories to ruminate upon.

Hypersensitivity and overactivity of the amygdala are at the core of anxiety-based disorders such as generalized anxiety disorder, phobias, PTSD, and other limbic-driven states that inhibit positive, rational (cortical) responses to stressors. Down-regulating amygdala reactivity and the resulting HPA axis stress-response cascade is of primary importance when treating clients suffering from fear-driven conditions. Cognitive therapeutic techniques are of little value to someone who cannot function cognitively (or "be cognitive"), so a bottom-up approach should be employed to bring the PFC back online, as it were. Creating an environment of safety and calm becomes the first step in helping the client regulate their amygdala reactivity. Allison and Rossouw (2013) describe the importance of a safe and controlled environment to effect change:

A therapeutic environment facilitates an enriched safe environment where psychotherapy has the potential to facilitate neural change and proliferation. Safety is essential for people in distress because it down-regulates the hypothalamus–pituitary adrenal system. When the fear response, which is triggered from the pons, amygdala, basal ganglia, hypothalamus, pituitary and adrenal glands, is activated, the distress activates the release of the corticotrophin releasing factor, adrenocorticotrophic hormone, adrenalin and cortisol. If these patterns are activated frequently, the patterns of firing will become well established, resulting in a default neural activation when a trigger is received. Through psychotherapy it is possible to facilitate down-regulation of the stress response system and encourage the development of new patterns of neural activation. Hence it is vital to enable change through the provision of a safe environment in which the individual can experience controlled incongruence, or stress, to prevent activation of the default distress response. A controlled environment is essential; however, if change is facilitated too quickly, the stress signal may be activated and the habitual pathological patterns facilitated. (p. 24)

THE HIPPOCAMPUS

The Hippocampus

The hippocampus is **another very important** structure in the limbic **system. It is involved in** the formation of declarative **memories that are** processed and transferred to neocortical areas through the process of memory consolidation and, notably, in the contextual anchoring of experience in time and space. The process of how the hippocampus transfers information to the neocortex to consolidate memory may be explained by what is called the hippocampal–neocortical dialogue. Structured interactions between the hippocampus and neocortex happen during slow-wave sleep, when sharp wave patterns dominate the hippocampus and there are bursts of neuron activity in synchrony with state changes in the cortex. This may be part of the process of consolidating memory into long-term state while you sleep.

Some researchers conceptualize the hippocampus not as a storage location for memory, but as a control centre that connects areas of the neocortex to activate the effective recall of memory. From this perspective we might think of the hippocampus as the brain's Google search engine, allowing fast and efficient searching of established memories in the neocortex to help assess and plan. A well-known function of the hippocampus is the capacity to learn and retrieve spatial memory: the what, when, and where qualities of an experience.

Hippocampus

Researchers have found that neurogenesis—the creation of new neurons—happens in the hippocampus with new learning. There is an upsurge of new neurons and associated circuits when a new task is learned, particularly in the case of physical tasks, and in enriched, stimulating environments. If the hippocampus is damaged, however, this can have significant effects on overall cognitive functioning, especially on spatial memory, and on explicit memory in general. Damage to the hippocampus can occur through prolonged exposure to stress hormones such as glucocorticoids (to which the hippocampus is particularly sensitive), highlighting the seriousness of chronic stress and its physiological impact. Basic feedback mechanisms in the hippocampus that help modulate the release of glucocorticoids during stress may be compromised, compounding the effects of chronic stress by leading to chronically elevated cortisol levels. It has been observed that some people suffering post-traumatic stress disorder (PTSD) have smaller hippocampal volume than the general population, and one study has found that this volume did not necessarily increase after therapy and symptom reduction (Lindauer et al., 2005). A compromised hippocampus may not anchor emotional reactions to a traumatic event to a specific time and space, and such reactions can reoccur inappropriately, as is typical in PTSD.

The hippocampus is also implicated in major depression, with findings of hippocampal volume being reduced as much as 8–19% in those with major depression, the reduction in volume being positively correlated with the duration of the depressive state. Similar correlations can be found with bipolar disorder and borderline personality disorder. It is possible that reduced hippocampal volume may be a risk factor rather than a consequence of chronic or excessive stress, so that individuals with a smaller hippocampus will be more prone to fear responses when exposed to traumatic events and less able to regulate that fear response (i.e., to keep the HPA axis stress-response cascade in check) and effectively integrate explicit and implicit memory of the trauma into long-term memory.

Much has been learned about the functions of the hippocampus through the study of a certain subject, Henry Gustav Molaison. Molaison, who in 1953 at the age of 27 had almost all of his hippocampus removed in an attempt to stop epileptic seizures, lost his ability to hold on to new semantic and episodic memories, being unable to consolidate them into long-term memory. He was able to remember what had happened a long time previously, and the older the memory the better he seemed to remember—just the opposite of what is normally observed. Molaison's general knowledge of the world (his semantic memory) was intact, but everything that happened after his surgery seemed new to him: he could only remember new experiences for a few seconds. Even the ability to recognize himself as he aged was lost, although he could recognize himself in old pictures. Interestingly, Henry was able to learn complex motor skills, and retain these skills (what we know as procedural or implicit memory), but was unable to remember learning them (declarative or explicit memory).

The left side hippocampus is represented here in blue. A compromised hippocampus may not anchor emotional reactions to a traumatic event to a specific time and space, and such reactions can reoccur inappropriately, as is typical in PTSD

THE HYPOTHALAMUS

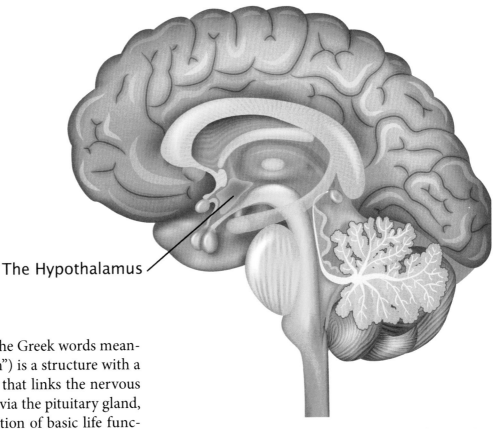

The Hypothalamus

T he hypothalamus (from the Greek words meaning "chamber underneath") is a structure with a variety of vital functions that links the nervous system to the endocrine system via the pituitary gland, for the regulation and coordination of basic life functions. The hypothalamus, as the name would suggest, is located below the thalamus and above the brainstem. It receives sensory inputs that detect changes in both internal and external environments. It receives direct inputs from smell, taste, visual, and somatosensory systems and also senses blood temperature, blood sugar, mineral levels, and a variety of hormones. The hypothalamus is closely connected to other limbic structures such as the hippocampus, amygdala, and cingulate cortex, and thus forms part of the continuum of emotional responsiveness. The medial zone of the hypothalamus is involved in motivated behaviours such as defensive behaviours.

The hypothalamus acts as a control centre for certain metabolic processes and activations of the autonomic nervous system involved in fluid and electrolyte balance, energy metabolism, circadian rhythms, sleep, fatigue, thirst, body temperature, hunger, attachment behaviours (including sexual and reproductive behaviour), to name a few. It synthesizes and secretes certain neurohormones that stimulate or inhibit the secretion of pituitary hormones.

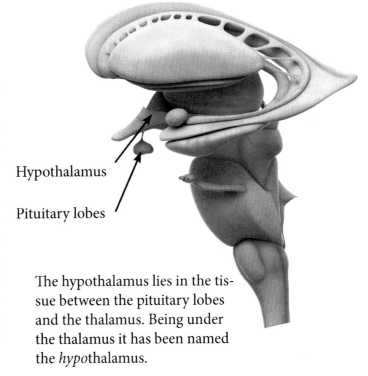

Hypothalamus

Pituitary lobes

The hypothalamus lies in the tissue between the pituitary lobes and the thalamus. Being under the thalamus it has been named the *hypo*thalamus.

The HPA Axis Response

The hypothalamic–pituitary–adrenal (HPA) axis response is the physiological mechanism that activates the body to respond to a threat. When a threat is detected by the amygdala, a physiological response is mediated through the hypothalamus–anterior pituitary gland. A neurohormone—corticotropin-releasing hormone (CRH) that has been manufactured in the paraventricular nucleus of the hypothalamus—triggers the anterior pituitary gland to release adrenocorticotropin hormone (ACTH) into the blood stream. The ACTH then triggers the release of glucocorticoids such as cortisol from the adrenal cortex above the kidneys. Feedback mechanisms in the hippocampus, hypothalamus and pituitary gland monitor the rising levels of cortisol in the blood and modulate the HPA axis stress-response cascade accordingly.

In the case where someone feels they are dealing with an extreme, uncontrollably stressful situation (such as the severe physical or sexual abuse of a child, or constant life-threatening situations as in war), the feedback mechanisms that dampen the HPA axis stress-response cascade can be damaged, and glucocorticoid levels continue to escalate. These excessive amounts of glucocorticoids can damage activated glutamate synapses and pyramidal cells in the hippocampus (where there are many glucocorticoid receptors), destabilizing previously formed neural connections and thus neural/mental function in the hippocampus. This may be positively correlated with the reduction in volume of the hippocampi of individuals who have suffered extreme stress and been diagnosed with PTSD.

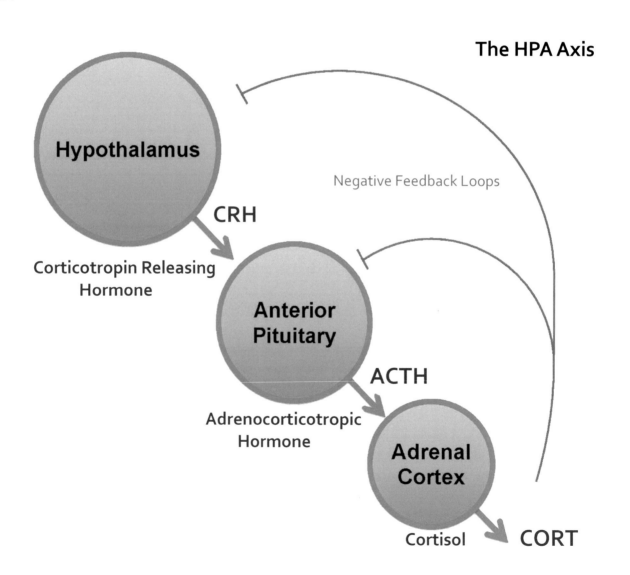

The HPA Axis

Hypothalamus

CRH

Corticotropin Releasing Hormone

Negative Feedback Loops

Anterior Pituitary

ACTH

Adrenocorticotropic Hormone

Adrenal Cortex

Cortisol CORT

Brian M Sweis - Wikimedia Commons

HPA Axis Response Pathway

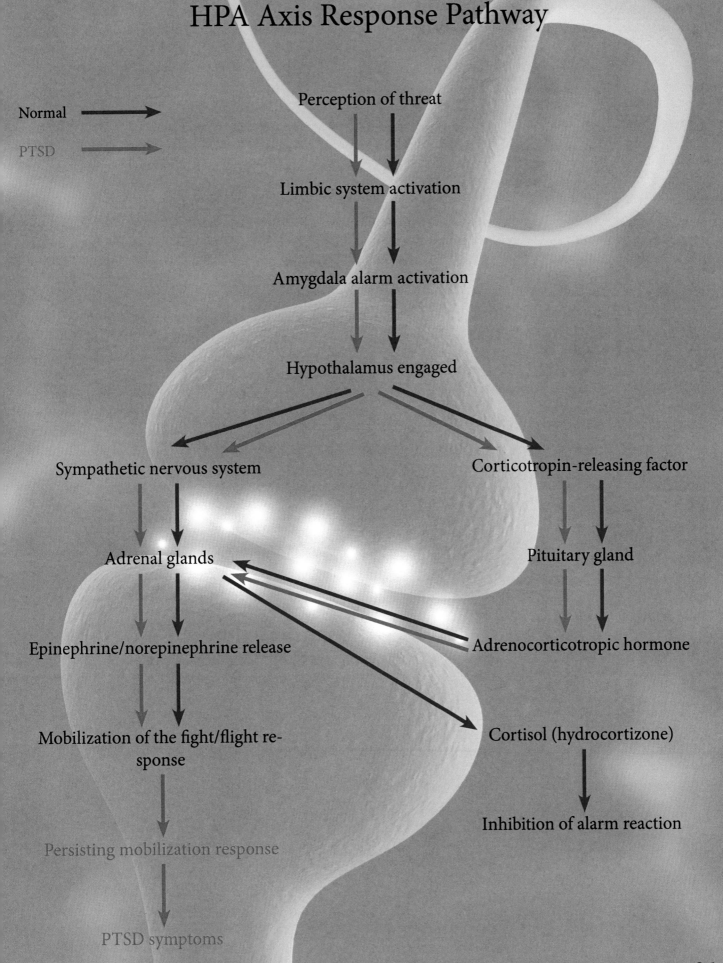

Normal →

PTSD →

Perception of threat

Limbic system activation

Amygdala alarm activation

Hypothalamus engaged

Sympathetic nervous system

Corticotropin-releasing factor

Adrenal glands

Pituitary gland

Epinephrine/norepinephrine release

Adrenocorticotropic hormone

Mobilization of the fight/flight response

Cortisol (hydrocortizone)

Persisting mobilization response

Inhibition of alarm reaction

PTSD symptoms

THE NEOCORTEX

The neocortex ("new bark") is composed of the topmost layers of the cerebral cortex, the part that is visible when looking at the external surface of the brain with all its folds and ridges. More than two thirds of the cerebral cortex is buried in grooves or fissures known as sulci: these folds give it a much greater surface area within the limited space of the skull. There are six layers to the neocortex, each layer about the thickness of a business card, and each functionally distinct. The layers consist of (and are linked by) vertical columns of neuronal clusters called "cortical columns". The communication between the columns and the layers allows for complex and sophisticated processing. It has been postulated that the top two layers provide an anticipatory function based on previous experience, and the bottom two layers attend to new information, while the middle two layers are devoted to forming a creative summation of the two (Hawkins & Blakeslee, 2004). It is also generally understood that the cortical columns in the left hemisphere are less cross-connected than those in the right; this correlates with the more connected and global view of the right hemisphere and the more linear and categorising view of the left. When we engage in the long-term practice of mindfulness—attending to sensations in the here and now—the bottom two layers of the neocortex are energized, adding thickness to the prefrontal cortex (PFC) and insula, at the same time shifting prefrontal activation toward the left side of the PFC, increasing the ability to be approach-oriented and reducing avoidance.

The Blue Brain Project (http://bluebrain.epfl.ch/) is an exciting multinational and multidisciplinary enterprise that is attempting to understand and model this complex system by building biologically detailed digital reconstructions and simulations of a rodent's brain– with the ultimate goal of doing the same for the human brain. The amount of computing power, together with the sheer size of the multidisciplinary team needed to grasp just a rudimentary understanding of these neural networks, attests to the sophistication and complexity of this system.

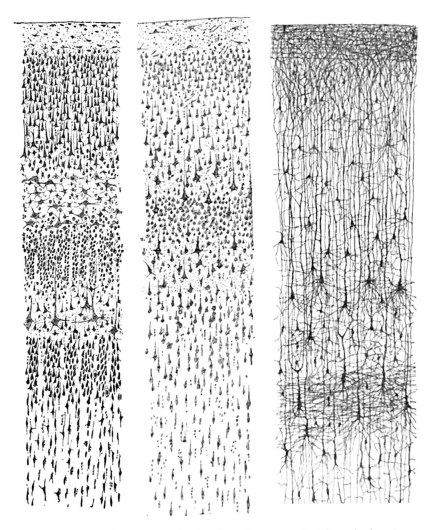

Above: Cortical lamination by Santiago Ramon y Cajal, each showing a vertical cross-section, with the surface of the cortex at the top. Left: Nissl-stained visual cortex of a human adult. Middle: Nissl-stained motor cortex of a human adult. Right: Golgi-stained cortex of a 1½-month-old infant. The Nissl stain shows the cell bodies of neurons; the Golgi stain shows the dendrites and axons of a random subset of neurons.

	molecular layer
	external granular layer
	layer of small and medium-sized pyramids
	internal granular layer
	ganglionic layer
	polymorphic cell layer
	white matter

A representative column of the neocortex with layers labeled.

MAJOR DIVISIONS

The neocortex has traditionally been divided in different ways to highlight various functional and structural areas. Here we will cover the broad strokes of functional areas, namely the occipital lobe, parietal lobes, temporal lobes, and the frontal lobes. But in any survey of the cortex, it is important to first acknowledge a widely used cortical map deriving from the work of German anatomist Korbinian Brodmann. Brodmann based his division of the cortex on the cytoarchitectural organization of the neurons, or the observation of how layers of neutrons look under a microscope after staining. Different areas of the cortex show specific patterns of cytoarchitecture, and thus a discrimination is made between different areas. Brodmann divided the cortex into 51 different areas and numbered them. Areas 1, 2, and 3 represent the primary somatosensory cortex, for example, while Area 10 is the anterior prefrontal cortex. Many texts and studies have used Brodmann's numbers to identify different areas of the cortex under discussion.

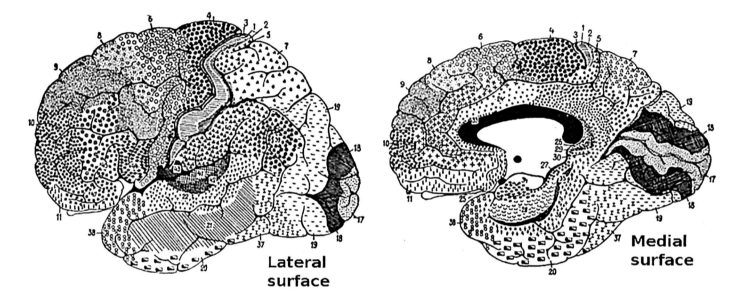

Lateral surface

Medial surface

Above: Regions of the human cerebral cortex delineated by Korvinian Brodman on the basis of cytoarchitecture. This image scanned and modified from the book *Anatomy of the Nervous System* by Stephen Walter Ranson & W. B. Saunders, 1920, p. 288.

Below: A 3D representation of Brodmann's areas by Mark Dow, research assistant at the Brain Development Lab at the University of Oregon.

Occipital lobe

Across the back of the brain is an area of the cerebrum—the occipital lobe—that is dedicated to processing visual information into meaningful chunks of perceptional material. The region is divided into a number of subregions, known as the primary visual cortex, the ventral stream, and the dorsal stream. The primary visual cortex processes low-level descriptions of orientation, spatial frequency and colour properties, whereas the ventral stream, sometimes called the "what" pathway, provides important information for the identification of stimuli, and the dorsal stream, sometimes called the "where" or "how" pathway, helps guide movement in response to outside stimuli.

It is worth noting that in borderline personality disorder there may be a deficit in the operation of the occipital lobe, leading to difficulties evaluating emotional facial expressions as well as other difficulties in processing visual information, which could lead to body dysmorphic disorder.

Image above showing dorsal stream (green) and ventral stream (purple) in the human brain visual system. (https://commons.wikimedia.org/wiki/File:Ventral-dorsal_streams.svg)

Parietal lobes

The parietal lobes play a major role in sensory processing and integrating information such as spatial/navigational sense, touch, and language, and the dorsal stream of the visual system. These lobes help us to become oriented and to establish an understanding of where we are in space. They also have a role in helping us understand speech and comprehending other sensory input.

Temporal lobes

Processing and integrating information about smells and sounds (such as recognising the sounds of one's language), and how these relate to our memory and emotions, is the domain of the temporal lobes. Closely associated with the hippocampus, the temporal lobes play a part in the formation of explicit long-term memory. The primary auditory cortex is situated within the left temporal lobe and processes the semantics of speech and vision: speech comprehension, naming, and verbal memory.

Frontal lobes

The frontal lobes are probably of most interest to psychotherapy because they are home to the PFC, an area vitally involved in executive functions such as concentration, organization, judgement, reasoning, decision-making, creativity, emotional regulation, social–relational abilities, and abstract thinking—in other words, all the functionality we rely on for healthy relationships with ourselves and others. We will look at the PFC separately because of its special importance to psychotherapy; however, the frontal lobes in general regulate voluntary movement, the retention of non-task-based memories that are often associated with emotions, dopamine-driven attention, reward motivations, and planning, to name just a few.

The Prefrontal Cortex

The PFC is the part of the cerebrum that lies directly behind the eyes and the forehead. More than any other part of the brain, this area dictates our personality, our goals, and our values. When we have a long-term goal, for example, which we are pursuing with value-congruent action, we maintain a neural representation of that goal so as to not be distracted or influenced by competing goals or alternate values (Grawe, 2007). If the PFC is damaged, it affects our personalities and the ability to orient our behaviour in line with our values and goals. The PFC is vital to the sense of self and others necessary for healthy interpersonal relationships and decision making.

As in the case of so many discoveries in neuroscience, we often learn what a brain area can do when it becomes damaged in some way. Phineas Gage was a young, reflective, determined, and goal-oriented man who, despite his youth, had been promoted to foreman on an American railroad construction project. But in an unfortunate accident on September 13, 1848, an explosion drove a tamping rod up through the left side of his face and out the top of his head. The rod passed through and destroyed much of his left PFC. Amazingly, Gage survived, and was even speaking within minutes of the accident. He was still conscious and talking to a physician about half an hour later, having introduced himself saying, "Doctor, here is business enough for you." Following his recovery, an early observation of a change in Gage's personality was noted by Dr. John Harlow:

> The equilibrium or balance, so to speak, between his intellectual faculties and animal propensities,

PREFRONTAL CORTEX

DORSOLATERAL PREFRONTAL CORTEX

ORBITOFRONTAL PREFRONTAL CORTEX

VENTROMEDIAL PREFRONTAL CORTEX

seems to have been destroyed. He is fitful, irreverent, indulging at times in the grossest profanity (which was not previously his custom), manifesting but little deference for his fellows, impatient of restraint or advice when it conflicts with his desires, at times pertinaciously obstinate, yet capricious and vacillating, devising many plans of future operations, which are no sooner arranged than they are abandoned in turn for others appearing more feasible. A child in his intellectual capacity and manifestations, he has the animal passions of a strong man. Previous to his injury, although untrained in the schools, he possessed a well-balanced mind, and was looked upon by those who knew him as a shrewd, smart business man, very energetic and persistent in executing all his plans of operation. In this regard his mind was radically changed, so decidedly that his friends and acquaintances said he was "no longer Gage". (Harlow, 1869, pp. 13-14)

Clearly, some important functions of Gage's personality had been altered by his injuries, although he did become more functional and socially adaptable as the years went on. Given a structured environment in which clear sequencing of tasks was part of the rehabilitation, Gage managed to retrain his brain to regulate itself in reference to values and goals.

The left and right sides of the PFC have different biases, with the left side oriented more toward approach, positive goals, and emotions, and the right side specialized more in avoidance and negative emotions. It is also worth noting that the left side of the PFC hosts more dopamine receptors/activity (associated with motivation and reward), while the right has greater norepinephrine activity (associated with anxiety). Individuals who appear to have a bias toward positive emotions may have a more activated left PFC, whereas right PFC activation is correlated with more negative emotional experiences. Any suggestion of a clear binary division is an oversimplification, as the experience of positive or negative emotions does not hinge purely on left/right PFC activation, but there is nonetheless evidence of a strong correlation. In studies of the neural correlates of depression, it has been found that left PFC activity is underactive relative to right PFC activity. It seems that less access to the positive bias of the left PFC may make it more difficult for the depressed individual to engage in positive goal-oriented thought and behaviour. Similarly,

the left PFC is more responsive to rewards than the right PFC, which is more responsive to punishment. Studies have found that the depressed individual is generally more sensitive to what may be perceived as punishment and does not respond as well to rewards. Moreover, the relative underactivation of the whole PFC in depressed individuals could account for them having less motivation for planning, problem solving, creativity, and so forth. In depression, not only is there underactivation of the PFC, but its volume has been found to be reduced as well. A depressed person with an underactive PFC of reduced volume is not going to demonstrate the rational problem solving abilities of someone without such deficits—the neural integrity to support such resilience is simply not there. This is where the active, approach-oriented and positively biased PFC of a therapist can be of great value to the depressed client. We will discuss the supportive right brain-to-right brain activity of therapy further when we address specific psychopathologies.

The PFC has been divided into a number of functionally distinct regions, described below.

Dorsolateral prefrontal cortex (DLPFC). The DLPFC is the topmost part of the PFC and is considered to

1868 diagram of Phineas Gage's skull and the damaged caused by the tamping rod – by John M. Harlow

have overall management of cognitive processes such as planning, cognitive flexibility, and working memory. This is an area specialising in problem solving and how to direct and maintain attention to a task. When we are focused on what is happening now, our working memory is engaged with the DLPFC and connecting with the hippocampus for the retrieval and consolidation of long-term explicit memories. A dysfunction in this area may lead to problems with working memory, processing in the hippocampus, and long-term memory, as well as the integration of verbal expression with emotions. Such memory deficits have been associated with PTSD due to an underactive left DLPFC. Other DLPFC deficits can manifest as a lack of spontaneity and affect (flat rather than negative), and attention deficit—due to an inability to maintain sufficient attention to see a task through to completion. In obsessive–compulsive disorder (which we will consider separately in a later section the DLPFC plays an important role in strengthening attentional skills to momentarily break the compulsion circuit and give the orbitofrontal cortex a chance to inhibit the runaway activation of the amygdala. As with many brain regions, there are significant hemispherical differences within the dorsolateral prefrontal cortex, the left DLPFC being associated with approach behaviours and the right with more avoidant behaviours.

Orbitofrontal cortex (OFC). The OFC, like the DLPFC, is involved in the cognitive processing of decision making; however, because of its close connection with the limbic system, it is particularly associated with our ability to make decisions based on emotional information. The OFC also plays a major role in forming social attachments and regulating emotions. This region can be thought of as a convergence zone for sensory and emotional information, effectively integrating external and internal worlds. Social information is processed and used to guide

us in our perceptions and interactions, and the OFC plays an important role in the interpretation of these complex social interactions, including, for example, the ability to understand a joke. The OFC may help us predict the reactions of others and modulate our behaviour accordingly. When there is a dysfunction in the orbitofrontal cortex, the normal cortical–subcortical modulation is not optimal—as is likely the case in borderline personality disorder (Schore, 2012). As with other areas of the PFC, the OFC has hemispherical differences. The left OFC is associated with positive emotions, while the right OFC is associated with more negative emotions.

Ventromedial prefrontal cortex (vmPFC). This part of the PFC helps us make decisions based on the bigger picture gathered from connections to the amygdala, temporal lobe, ventral segmental area, olfactory system, and the thalamus. It is very well connected, receiving and sending a lot of information that influences many brain regions, including the amygdala. The vmPFC plays an important role with the OFC in regulating our emotions, especially in social situations. It is also vital for personal and social decision making and the ability to learn from our mistakes. Our capacity to make judgements and allow our emotions to assist in decision making is mediated by this region of the brain. Activation of the vmPFC is also associated with courage, suppression of negative emotions, compassion, shame, and guilt.

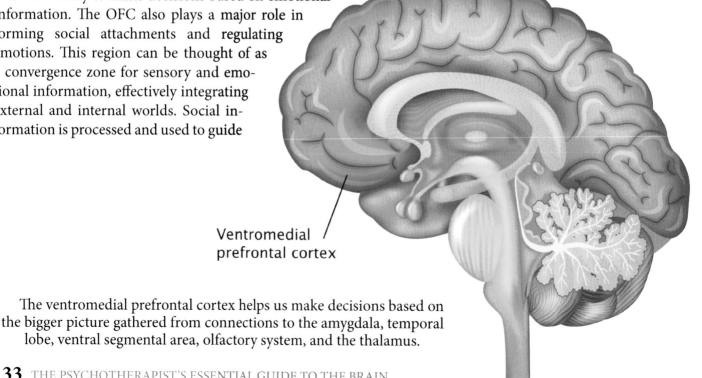

Ventromedial
prefrontal cortex

The ventromedial prefrontal cortex helps us make decisions based on the bigger picture gathered from connections to the amygdala, temporal lobe, ventral segmental area, olfactory system, and the thalamus.

PHRENOLOGY

German neuroanatomist and physiologist Franz Joseph Gall (1758–1828) was a pioneer in efforts to determine the location of functions on the cortex of the brain. The discipline, which became known as phrenology, was very popular in the 19th century, with the Edinburgh Phrenological Society established in 1820.

Phrenologists would feel the surface of the skull to determine the size of the underlying brain region. Each discrete region, it was believed, had a unique function. Gall claimed there were 27 such regions, or "organs", and that by feeling an individual's skull, he could determine the character of the person from any enlargements or indentations. Apparently, early phrenologists believed there was a direct correlation between skull topography and cortical function.

Elaborate maps were drawn identifying the different "brain organs" under specific areas of the skull, and using this reference the phrenologist could determine the character, strengths, and weaknesses of any individual on the basis of what areas were pronounced.

The idea had a forerunner in Johann Kaspar Lavater (1741–1801), a Swiss pastor, who believed that an individual's character and mind were revealed by their external frame—a concept he termed physiognomy. In his book *The Pocket Lavater, or, The Science of Physiognomy* (1832), Lavater stated:

> The various thoughts which arise in the mind, the different passions which agitate the soul of man, are respectively connected with his features and the external parts of his frame; and so intimate is their correspondence, that the expression of the countenance, more rapid than speech, betrays his sentiments and emotions, and gives to his utterance energy and animation. The one was designed as a mirror in which we might behold the other reflected. (p. 15)

He later gave examples such as "Of the forehead, when the forehead is perfectly perpendicular, from the hair to the eyebrows, it denotes an utter deficiency of understanding" (Lavater, 1832, p. 24).

Other books were written on how to recognize idiots and intellectuals, criminals and those with good moral character. Phrenologists made diagnoses about people's motives, abilities, temperaments, while talent spotters used phrenology to identify people best suited for a job.

At the beginning of the 20th century, rising interest in evolution and anthropology sparked renewed interest in phrenology. Attention was drawn to the evolving shape of the human skull through the influential work of Paul Bouts, who considered that the prehistoric skull shape was prevalent in criminals and savages. Some Europeans even attempted to recruit the idea as scientific proof of their superiority over "lesser" races, with theories appearing about Caucasians being the most beautiful and civilized peoples in contrast to such as the Australian Aborigines and Maoris, who were considered—purely on the basis of their outward appearance—to have less "elevated" brains. Such ideas were later discredited as pseudoscience.

In the Victorian era, when phrenology was taken very seriously, gender stereotyping was also empowered by this "science", which served as a justification for denying women participation in politics and citizenship (Staum, 2003). McCandless (1992) notes that as a source of psychological insight, phrenology drew thousands to consult specialists for advice on matters as diverse as hiring employees and finding a marriage partner.

NEUROCHEMICALS

We know the brain is a complexity of neural networks, and the pathways of these networks describe thinking patterns. But that is only half the story, since the networks themselves cannot work without the electrochemical action of neurotransmitters. A synergy exists between established neural pathways and the activation of these pathways, which is mediated by neurochemicals. As therapists, we want to know what we can do in practice to enhance positive (i.e., helpful) neurochemical activity and, likewise, what it is that inhibits or dysregulates such activity, without reverting to pharmacology. Therefore, a basic understanding of the specific neurochemicals that modulate the nervous system is essential to understanding what drives certain pathologies, why certain interventions are effective, and why some are not.

There are two main groups of neurotransmitters to consider: those that act slowly and bring about enduring changes, and those that act quickly and have a more temporary effect on brain activity. The fast-acting neurotransmitters are amino acids, the most prominent of these being glutamate, aspartate, glycine, and gamma-aminobutyric acid (GABA). Glutamate, aspartate, and glycine come from the proteins we consume, and GABA comes from a simple modification of glutamate. The slower-acting neurotransmitters are biogenic amines.

Serotonin (above) is involved in the regulation of mood, appetite, and sleep, as well as memory and learning. It is considered a major antidepressant based on a theory of depression revolving around serotonin levels.

Melatonin (below) helps regulate our circadian rhythm (day/night cycles). As melatonin levels rise we become sleepy. Interestingly, the nightly release of melatonin is typically delayed as children become teenagers, leading to later sleeping and waking times. Melatonin is also a powerful antioxidant.

Amino Acids

Glutamates. Glutamates act as excitatory neurotransmitters in the brain and are essential to normal functioning. Receptor sites are either the fast-acting ionotropic types such as AMPA (i.e., α-amino-3-hydroxy-5-methyl-4-isoxazole propionic acid), which primarily activate or inhibit, or the slower acting N-methyl D-aspartate (NMDA) types, which facilitate a strengthening of the synaptic connection known as long-term potentiation. Glutamates bind with activating receptors (AMPA), resulting in fast activation of the postsynaptic neuron.

Gamma-aminobutyric acid (GABA). GABA is an inhibitory neurotransmitter that plays counterpart to glutamates: if glutamate is the accelerator of the brain, GABA is the brake. There is an obvious need in an active system of this kind to modulate and balance activation with a dampening or braking system, and this is where GABA comes into its own. It acts quickly, binding with GABA receptors to produce an inhibiting effect on the postsynaptic cell. GABA and AMPA interactions are seen across the brain and result in much of the fast action of our neural processes, including many of our thought processes and much of our sensory input/processing.

Monoamines

The monoamines are slower-acting and more localized in distribution than the amino acids, and are known to be released from non-synaptic sites. Monoamines are synthesized from a single amino acid (hence *mono-amine*). There are two broad groups of monoamines: catecholamines and indolamines. Among the catecholamines are dopamine, epinephrine, and norepinephrine, all synthesized from tyrosine, which is then converted to L-dopa and dopamine (see Figure 1). Among the indolamines are serotonin (5-hydroxytryptamine, or 5-HT) and melatonin.

Catecholamines. Catecholamines trigger physiological changes to prepare the body for physical activity such as the fight-or-flight response.

Dopamine. Dopamine has many functions, including motivation, arousal, reinforcement, reward, motor control, and executive function. From a therapeutic point of view we can equate reward with dopamine, be it appetite or sexual satisfaction, or even complex social and cognitive satisfactions (such as understanding what is going on in your client's brain!). Most dopaminergic neurons are in the midbrain and hypothalamus.

Norepinephrine and epinephrine. Norepinephrine and epinephrine have dual functions as hormones and neurotransmitters. They play a part in the fight-or-flight

Figure 1. Synthesis of catecholamines

response (see The Neurochemistry of Stress below). Norepinephrine is produced by certain neurons as well as the adrenal glands, but epinephrine is only produced by the adrenal glands. Norepinephrine is a psychoactive molecule in the brain, promoting blood circulation to the skeletal muscles. Epinephrine is not a psychoactive compound, but increases energy production via glucose release in response to rising norepinephrine levels.

Dopamine has many functions, including motivation, arousal, reinforcement, reward, motor control, and executive function.

Melatonin helps regulate our circadian rhythm (day/night cycles). As melatonin levels rise we become sleepy.

It also relaxes muscles to dilate the bronchial tubes and allow increased oxygen intake. Epinephrine and norepinephrine were called adrenaline and noradrenaline until the brand name Adrenaline was registered by a drug company. Somewhat confusingly, neurons releasing norepinephrine are still called "noradrenergic" and those releasing epinephrine "adrenergic".

Indolamines. The indolamines comprise a family of neurotransmitters that includes serotonin and melatonin (derived from serotonin).

5-HT. 5-HT (serotonin) is involved in the regulation of mood, appetite, and sleep, as well as memory and learning. It is considered a major antidepressant in a theory of depression revolving around serotonin levels.

Melatonin. Melatonin helps regulate our circadian rhythm (day/night cycles). As melatonin levels rise we become sleepy. Interestingly, the nightly release of melatonin is typically delayed as children become teenagers, leading to later sleeping and waking times. Melatonin is also a powerful antioxidant

The monoamine hypothesis of depression postulates that a lack of serotonin flow in the brain leads to symptoms of depression (as well as anxiety, obsessions, and compulsions). One of the chemical solutions that has been engineered is that of serotonin reuptake inhibition. The serotonin that is released into the synaptic cleft (the space between a neuron's axon and a neighbouring dendrite) is recaptured by the presynaptic cell through a reuptake mechanism that recycles serotonin in the cell. A selective serotonin reuptake inhibitor (SSRI) will block the reuptake mechanism to preserve more serotonin in the synaptic cleft, so that more of the chemical is available to connect to the neighbouring dendrite.

Acetylcholine

Acetylcholine (ACh) is another small-molecule neurotransmitter that is used by motor neurons of the nervous system (at the neuromuscular junction) to activate muscles. Neurons releasing ACh are known as cholinergic. ACh also plays a role in the autonomic nervous system and in the central nervous system, where it modulates plasticity, arousal, reward, enhancement of sensory perceptions, and sustained attention. ACh is involved in memory and learning: memory can be enhanced when drugs are used to increase the activity of ACh in the brain. Disruption of

Small-Molecule Neurotransmitters		
Class	Subclass	Neurotransmitter
Amino acids		glutamate aspartate glycine GABA
Monoamines	catecholamines	dopamine epinephrine norepinephrine
	indolamines	serotonin
Acetylcholine		acetylcholine
Unconventional neurotransmitters	soluble gasses (gasotransmitters)	nitric oxide carbon monoxide hydrogen sulfide
	endocannabinoids	anandamide
Large-Molecule Neurotransmitters		
Neuropeptides	pituitary peptides hypothalamic peptides brain-gut peptides opioid peptides miscellaneous peptides	

ACh neurotransmission can disrupt memory, as in the case of the neurodegenerative disease Alzheimer's.

"Unconventional" Neurotransmitters

There are a few classes of what are known as "unconventional" neurotransmitters. We will consider two of these: soluble gases (or gasotransmitters) and endocannabinoids. Soluble gases such as nitric oxide and carbon monoxide pass through cell membranes and stimulate the production of second messengers before being deactivated when they are converted to other molecules. In some synapses, these soluble gases perform what is known as retrograde transmission, delivering a feedback signal from the postsynaptic neuron to the presynaptic neuron (seemingly to regulate the presynaptic neuron). Anandamide (*N*-arachidonoylethanolamine, or AEA) belongs to the endocannabinoid class of neurotransmitters. AEA is a fatty acid neurotransmitter that has effects in both the central and the peripheral nervous system. Much is still unknown about this neurotransmitter, but it has been shown to play a role in the regulation of feeding behaviour, and also in motivation, pleasure, and reward. Its name comes from the Sanskrit *ananda* ("joy, bliss, delight") and amide (an acid).

Neuropeptides

In addition to the small-molecule neurotransmitters described above, there is a large group (over 100) of protein-like, large-molecule neurotransmitters known as neuropeptides, which can be grouped into the following categories: pituitary peptides (first identified as pituitary hormones), hypothalamic peptides (first identified as hypothalamus hormones), brain–gut peptides (first identified in the gut), opioid peptides (with a similar chemical structure to opium), and miscellaneous peptides (as a catch-all for the rest). Peptides will often coexist and act with other neurotransmitters, but they have much more diverse effects, such as gene expression, local blood flow, synaptogenesis, and changes in glial cells. These actions tend to be prolonged and can have significant effects on behaviour.

THE NEUROCHEMISTRY OF STRESS

In 1914, the physiologist Walter Cannon named the sympathetic response to a threat the "fight or flight" response. As we have observed, the chemical response to this fight-or-flight response is known as the hypothalamic–pituitary–adrenal (HPA) axis response.

When we perceive a threat, the corticotropin-releasing hormone (CRH) is released from the hypothalamus together with beta endorphins. CRH is produced in the paraventricular nucleus (PVN) of the hypothalamus, and this triggers the release of adrenocorticotropin hormone (ACTH) in the pituitary gland. Interestingly, CRH will also inhibit the secretion of reproductive hormones and subsequent reproductive functions. The beta-endorphin release from the hypothalamus plays a role in pain reduction and stimulates the release of epinephrine from the adrenal medulla. Vasopressin is also released from the PVN, and this plays a role in regulating blood pressure and facilitates the release of ACTH.

ACTH flows from the pituitary gland into the bloodstream and releases the hormone cortisol from the adrenal cortex. (The adrenal glands sit above each kidney.) Levels of glucocorticoids like cortisol are closely monitored at each step of the HPA axis as a feedback mechanism to regulate the stress response. Cortisol increases blood-sugar levels, suppresses the immune system, and increases metabolism. Because high levels of cortisol suppress the immune system—the assumption being that the suppression helps to protect against an overactivation of the immune system and minimize inflammatory tissue damage—it has been observed that high levels of cortisol will lengthen wound healing time. As in the monitoring of glucocorticoids to modulate the HPA-axis response, there is also a feedback loop involving the immune system in which certain cytokines can activate the HPA axis.

When the HPA axis is set in motion by a perceived threat, or an exaggerated fear of something that is not an actual, physical threat, the physiological response can be taxing and potentially damaging to the body. Chronically raised glucocorticoid levels not only increase blood-sugar levels and suppress the immune system but also inhibit learning, because new neural connections in the hippocampus are damaged, and even previously established memory retrieval is inhibited.

EPIGENETICS

The mature brain was once thought immutable, until evidence began to accumulate that it was, in fact, somewhat malleable. Now the remarkable plasticity of the brain is common knowledge. Similarly we have undergone a paradigm shift in our thinking about DNA. We now know that DNA is not fixed—in fact it is also quite malleable, and genes are as capable of modification as the brain. Both the brain and our genetic make-up have a level of plasticity that allows wiring pathways and gene expression to change with experience over time. This is illustrated by the case of genetically identical twins, who have obvious DNA-driven similarities, yet also differences that develop in response to personal experience (Kaminsky et al., 2009).

DNA, the molecule that acts as long-term storage for our genetic information, is also capable of regulating its own use. Most of our DNA is in fact not dedicated to the primary role of protein production. This non-protein-coding DNA was believed for years to be relatively useless, even acquiring the moniker "junk DNA". We are only now discovering that junk DNA performs a number of important functions, and that RNA strands (ribonucleic acid transcribed from certain non-coding DNA) act to regulate, stimulate, and disrupt the activity of protein production. Much of this is an epigenetic response: in other words, it is dependent on the nature of the individual's experience in the context of particular environmental conditions. This discovery represents an enormous breakthrough in our understanding of our malleable biology.

Epigenetics (literally "above the genes"), also known as behavioural epigenetics, is the study of how environmental factors influence gene expression both within and through heritable changes in DNA. The environment can "mark" genes, dramatically or subtly, changing levels of expression either transiently or for a lifetime—even to subsequent generations (Peckham, 2013). It is the mechanism by which genes adapt to the environment, shaping gene expression to best adapt to whatever circumstances confront us.

When the environment prompts heritable changes in gene expression, no changes are made to the underlying DNA sequence (Levenson & Sweatt, 2005). In any strand of DNA, only a well-defined portion of the genetic possibilities within the DNA are expressed, and the rest are permanently, semi-permanently, or temporarily turned off. To use the language of geneticists, the universal DNA genotype is epigenetically changed to a cell-specific phenotype. The detail of epigenetic ac-

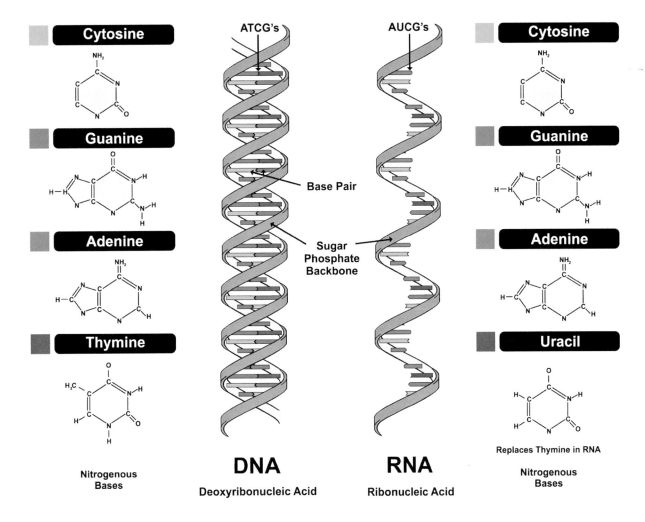

Cytosine

Guanine

Adenine

Thymine

Nitrogenous Bases

DNA
Deoxyribonucleic Acid

ATCG's

Base Pair

Sugar Phosphate Backbone

AUCG's

RNA
Ribonucleic Acid

Cytosine

Guanine

Adenine

Uracil

Replaces Thymine in RNA

Nitrogenous Bases

tion is complex, but the principle is quite straightforward. By adding or subtracting chemicals, it is possible to "silence" a gene and thus make it impossible for that gene to be expressed in that cell or in any of its daughter cells. This is not exactly the same process we refer to as "turning genes on and off", which is more about utilizing genes that are readily available in accordance with particular needs at the time. Genes that are epigenetically silenced are taken completely out of the picture (Hill, 2013).

One way that a gene is silenced is when chemical alterations are made to tiny chemical tails that emerge from each of the eight histones (proteins that act as spools around which DNA winds and becomes compact). Addition or subtraction of these chemicals allows or disallows transcription factors to attach to the promoter region (the part of the DNA that starts the transcription of a particular gene). The process that has received the most attention is acetylation: when a histone tail is acetylated, the difference in ionic (electrochemical) charge between the histone and the section of DNA wrapped around it is neutralized (the larger the difference in charge between objects, the stronger the electromagnetic attraction). The effect of acetylation in neutralizing this difference is that the DNA is looser and therefore accessible to transcription factors. When the histone tail is de-acetylated, the difference in charge increases, causing the DNA to wrap tightly around the histone so that it is impossible for transcription to occur (Grunstein, 1997; for a general discussion of DNA methylation and histone modification, see Peckham, 2013).

Another, entirely different silencing mechanism is a change added to the DNA code itself. In particular positions, usually near the promoter region in the gene (at what is described as CpG nucleotides), the cytosine "letter" of the DNA code is methylated, which blocks the transcription factor from binding to the promoter region and, again, stops gene expression (Comb & Goodman, 1990). The crucial point here is that, through a series of intricate and elegant processes that evoke images of a symphony, the information in our genes is constantly being brought into activity or silenced.

Studies of rats and their maternal behaviour have demonstrated that the quality of maternal care of rat pups in the first weeks of life influences the patterns of gene expression that affect social engagement and self-defence (Kauffman & Meaney, 2007). The pups that received enriched stimulation from their mothers showed different patterns of gene expression in their hippocampus, prefrontal cortex, and amygdala from the pups who did not get as much maternal care. Subsequently, the well-cared-for rats demonstrated better social skills and were more approach-oriented in their environment and less fearful (Baylin, 2013). One of the most notable differences observed in the well-cared-for rat pups was the development of a robust stress-response system. The reason for this is that the hippocampus has corticosterone stress-hormone receptors that help turn off this system after a stressful experience. These receptors were more highly expressed in the well-cared-for rats, who were able to down-regulate the stress response faster than their not-so-well-cared-for peers. The nurturing contributed to less self-defensiveness in these individuals and more exploration and social connectedness.

The research with rats has since been extended to primates and humans, to investigate the extent of gene expression as a result of environmental factors, especially attachment factors. Interestingly, the human studies on levels of care and epigenetic effects show a striking parallel to the rodent studies, suggesting that all sorts of early childhood experiences (and even pre-birth and birth factors such as Caesarean section) heighten the DNA methylation that negatively affects neurons and brain plasticity. Peckham (2013) says of these studies:

It is tempting to speculate that perhaps lower levels of care restrict the variety of genes that can be expressed, whereas higher levels of care are the epigenetic gateway to our available genome. We speak of wanting to give our children "every opportunity", but the reality of what epigenetic opportunities are available to our children could largely depend on the care we give them very early in life. Access to the widest potential of their genome could be profoundly influenced by their experience of our care, and if the genes that are accessed by enhanced care perform plasticity-related functions, the effect of that care is compounded for good or ill. Poor care may mean that fewer plasticity-related genes are expressed, thus restricting a child's (and the adult's) potential to learn, remember, or adapt within their environment, manifesting in less flexibility and perhaps more stereotyped or rigid responses. (p. 15)

Research suggests that early life experiences with attachment figures activate different patterns of gene expression—but that experience-dependent gene expression is not limited to these early experiences and continues throughout life (Baylin, 2013). These findings have significant implications for psychotherapy. The adaptive role of epigenetic mechanisms is to ensure the young are well equipped to survive in the particular environments in which they find themselves. A safe and enriched environment, therefore, will help shape a healthy nervous system that connects with people, is approach-orientated, and is able to down-regulate fear responses quickly. In contrast, an unsafe and harsh environment will produce a nervous system that is epigenetically geared toward self-defence, avoidance, and an easily activated and prolonged stress response. The unfortunate outcome of this programming is a compromised system of self-regulation (in terms of the control mechanisms from the prefrontal cortex to the limbic system and a stress-response feedback mechanism to down-regulate an overly sensitive amygdala, to name just two), which can lead to a life of low self-esteem, avoidance, anxiety, and depression.

But are we to remain victims of our early childhood experiences forever, genetically speaking? Fortunately the answer is no. Just as we are learning that early experience shapes the development of neural networks, we are now learning that the early years are the most critical for the epigenetic shaping of our brains; but similarly, just as the plasticity of neural networks opens them to transformation via new experiences and memory reconsolidation, so we are discovering that our genetic expressions are open to change in response to perceived changes in our environment. Furthermore, not only are epigenetic processes associated with social and emotional factors, they are also associated with exercise, sleep/wake cycles, mindfulness practices, and diet. This opens up for psychotherapists a whole new world of hope for change, and a more integrative model of mental-health intervention.

Pharmacotherapeutics is making inroads into reversing epigenetic marks caused by environmental experiences on genes associated with stress response and mental well-being. But for those who are looking for an alternative to pharmacology, the enriched environment of safety, social connectedness, and sensory/motor/cognitive stimulation can have a mitigating effect on the negative epigenetic processes of the early years. As Peckham (2013) notes:

> Environmental enrichment is a powerful tool to effect epigenomic changes, which subsequently affect the levels of BDNF and modulate HPA axis activity, which, in turn, builds resilience to, or delays the onset of, various psychiatric or neurodegenerative disorders. . . . Psychotherapy can be seen as a form of emotional environmental enrichment. It is perfectly placed to offer an enriched experience of a caring relationship, albeit an asymmetrical one, where one can receive empathic, attuned attention that may be wholly novel and life changing. By offering a new, benevolent experience of relationship, psychotherapy can be reasonably assumed to change gene expression, calming a hyperreactive stress axis and ameliorating the effects of an epigenetically scarred BDNF promoter, and in so doing, changing our responses to stress and, perhaps, our capacity to learn and flexibly respond to emotionally challenging situations. For the client in psychotherapy—as in many situations in life—it really is the experience that counts. (p. 17)

Brain plasticity has revolutionized our thinking about the capacity to make positive changes in our lives. Epigenetics is one way the body "writes down" and memorizes ongoing life experience in a way that helps us adapt to our experiences. Ultimately, what we do, when we do it, and how we feel about it while we are doing it all contribute to the way experience assembles and shapes the building materials in our DNA to construct the person that we see both in the bathroom mirror and in the mirror of our friends and loved ones. But what in childhood served as adaptive programming may no longer be appropriate to our needs and environment in adulthood, and so we can and should change. It is exciting to know that we have the capacity to change our neural networks, our emotional memory, and our mental schemas. And with a little help, we can even change the expression of our genes to better adapt to our current circumstances.

MOTIVATION

THE PSYCHOTHERAPIST'S ESSENTIAL GUIDE TO THE BRAIN

In 1988, French neurologist Michel Habib and colleague Michel Poncet became intrigued by stories of people who would, all of a sudden, lose their motivation and interest in life. For example, a 64-year-old retired police officer had suddenly become apathetic, inactive and prostrate. He was admitted to the neurology ward a few weeks after the onset of behavioural changes and was assessed as having some muscle rigidity with decreased spontaneous movements, facial amimia, and a Parkinson's-like gait. His CT scan seemed normal for a patient of his age, but he displayed a dramatic decrease in spontaneous activity: he was unable to make plans and seemed to have no will or identifiable desires—not even a desire to eat or a preference for any particular foods. Moreover, when asked what was going on in his mind, there appeared to be no spontaneous mental activity, yet he was fully conscious and orientated. When questioned about his mood, he said he wasn't sad, depressed, or anxious.

Another very similar case involved a 60-year-old university professor, highly respected in his field, who also displayed a dramatic decrease in activity and motivation, according to family and peers. His neurological exam identified a moderate slowing of movements and poor spontaneous verbal expression. For someone who had been a highly active professional, he was surprisingly unconcerned by his sudden loss of motivation. His relatives described him as having been energetic, motivated, and highly invested in both his work and leisure activities, such as gardening, reading, and fine cuisine. Something dramatic had happened to this man. The radical change in his motivation and demeanour persisted and was observed again at a 7-year follow-up. He described his condition in these words:

I just lack spirit, energy . . . I have no go. I must force myself to get up in the morning; I do things just because I ought to, without any liking or enthusiasm. I have no appetite or need for eating; I only eat by principle.

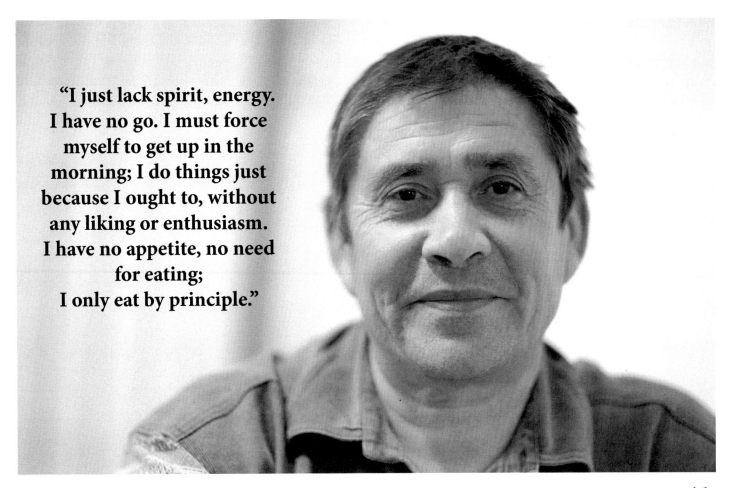

"I just lack spirit, energy. I have no go. I must force myself to get up in the morning; I do things just because I ought to, without any liking or enthusiasm. I have no appetite, no need for eating; I only eat by principle."

Coronal slices of human brain showing the striatum, and globus pallidus (GPe and GPi). White matter is shown in dark grey, grey matter is shown in light grey. Image Andrew Gillies, Wikimedia Commons

anything to say, he would typically respond with, "I'm just thinking of nothing . . . no idea, no question, no thought at all."

These and other similar cases, Habib would find, had in common injuries to regions of the basal ganglia: damage to either the striatum, by way of tiny pinpricks of burst vessels restricted to the caudate nuclei, or the globus pallidus. After consideration of these cases and the neurological evidence, Habib went on to formulate a model of a cortical–subcortical loop involved in converting motivational processes into behaviour (Habib, 2004). He showed how the limbic (or ventral) striato-pallidal circuit he described received emotional information from the amygdala and hippocampus and projected that information to the rest of the basal ganglia involved in initiating and organizing motor acts (Habib, 2004).

Researcher Mauricio Delgado, who has studied the neural substrates recruited during decision-making, found that activity in the caudate nucleus increases when we have a choice. And having a choice, as Klaus Grawe identified in his consistency model (Grawe, 2007), equates to a sense of greater control. We could say that choice is the vehicle for exercising control (Leotti, Iyengar, Ochsner, 2010). Having a choice, then, is fundamentally motivating. In one study, Delgado and co-author Lauren Leotti stated that even "the anticipation of choice itself was associated with increased activity in corticostriatal regions, particularly the ventral striatum, involved in affective and motivational processes" (Leotti

He could carry out some professional tasks, but as a routine only, not because he had any motivation to do them. He would not initiate conversations; he was never bored, anxious, or depressed; and he never complained about anything. He still attended board meetings but was never the first to speak. He seemed to be shut up inside a profound passivity, unaware and unconcerned. When asked a question he would answer appropriately, but when asked about what he was thinking or if he had

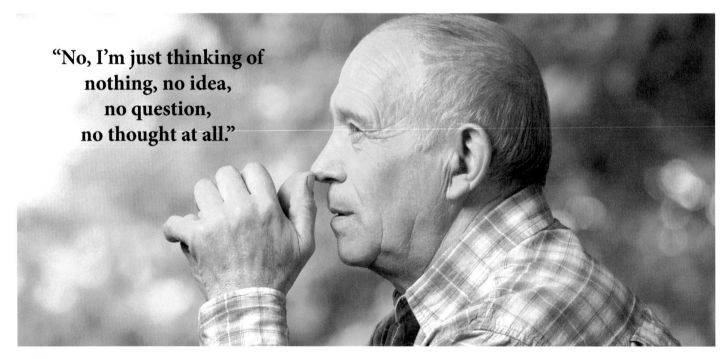

"No, I'm just thinking of nothing, no idea, no question, no thought at all."

& Delgado, 2011, p. 1310). Having a choice is preferable even if making a certain choice makes no real difference to the outcome—we simply prefer to have a sense of control. In an earlier study conducted with residents of a nursing home, Langer and Rodin (1976) found that the opportunity to exercise choice influenced subsequent mood, quality of life, and longevity.

Our well-being depends on our belief that we have some control over our day-to-day environment. Indeed, Leotti and colleagues would argue that it is a biological imperative (Leotti, Iyengar, & Ochsner, 2010). The neural substrate for this need for control is the corticostriatal network—the same network that was implicated in motivation (or the lack thereof) in Habib's cases. Neuroimaging studies have demonstrated that choice recruits circuits that are involved in reward and motivation processing, which in turn increases activity in the striatum. This increased activity might also reflect an increased motivational incentive when there is choice. As Leotti and colleagues suggested, "If free choice preferentially activates the striatum, a region involved in reward processing and goal-directed behavior, we might hypothesize that choice itself may be inherently rewarding" (Leotti, Iyengar, & Ochsner, 2010, p. 460).

From these studies emerges a theory of motivation: giving people choices provides them with a sense of autonomy and self-determination that is fundamentally motivating. Each of us from our own experience would know that it is difficult to feel motivated when there seemingly are no options available to us in the circumstances. But increase the opportunity for choice, and our corticostriatal network lights up, and we find ourselves a little more motivated. When we perceive there are choices we are capable of making, we start to sense an internal locus of control—that rewarding feeling that tells us we have a degree of self-determination.

The practical implications of this research are relatively simple. When considering clients who seem to have no motivation and are apathetic, it is advisable to look into their sense of control. It may be that they perceive they have very little control, that they have few choices, and that an external locus of control (a sense that the government, their boss, their mother is holding the strings) has stripped them of self-determination. Look for ways to encourage more corticostriatal network activity by introducing choices, even small ones, to help your client regain a sense of control and subsequent motivation.

Our well-being depends on our belief that we have some control over our day-to-day environment. Indeed, Leotti and colleagues would argue that it is a biological imperative

MIRROR NEURONS

I talian neuroscientists in the mid-1990s were studying the premotor areas of the frontal lobes of monkeys when they discovered a remarkable connection between the firing of neurons in the motor cortex and visual perception (Gallese et al., 1996). While monitoring a neuron that had been activated when a monkey ate a peanut, researchers noticed that the same neuron was activated when the monkey simply saw the researcher eat a peanut. It was as if the motor neuron was "mirroring" what the monkey saw. Perception and action were seen to be linked in a way that had not previously been understood. As it turned out, some of these mirroring neurons where highly specific in their response to visual perception—such as only firing at the perception of picking up a banana with the right hand or peeling it with the thumb and forefinger (Rizzolatti & Arbib, 1998). Much research on mirror neurons has been conducted since this serendipitous finding, resulting in a deeper understanding of the social nature of our own minds.

Mirror neurons have both motor and perceptual function, and respond to acts that are perceived to carry purpose or intention. Mirror neurons will not "mirror" behaviour unless there is a predictable sequence based on intention—like the scientist bringing a peanut up to his mouth as opposed to randomly waving his hands around. The observing monkey knows from experience what bringing a peanut up to one's mouth is all about and can anticipate the ensuing sensation of putting the peanut into his mouth: the mirror system has learnt by experience.

Extending the study of mirror neurons from monkey to human, Marco Iacoboni and colleagues suggested that mirror neurons help us understand the intentional state of others (Carr, Iacoboni, Dubeau, Maziotta, & Lenzi, 2003). The basic premise is that our perception of another person's predictable movements helps us understand what is going on in their mind. Although single-cell recordings of mirror neurons in human subjects would be too invasive for research purposes, much can be surmised from the work with monkeys and less invasive scanning of human subjects (such as EEG, MEG, fMRI, and TMS; see Ramachandran, 2011, pp. 141–142). Iacoboni and colleagues found an integrated system that includes mirror neurons in the frontal and parietal cortex, which coordinated with the superior temporal region to form a neural image of the mental state of another—the foundation of empathic attunement. These areas are at the intersection of inner and outer experience, representing a convergence of visual, motor, and emotional processing (Iacoboni et al., 2001). Cozolino (2014) put it this way:

The frontal lobes, especially in the left hemisphere, ground us in time through action plans, means–goals relationships, and a memory for the future. The parietal lobes, especially in the right, construct three-dimensional space, the context within which our real and imagined actions take place. And since our actions contain both purpose and context, human experience emerges from within the interwoven matrix of "space–time" constructed by the synergy of these two executive networks. (p. 212)

It is thought that mirror neurons' capacity to internally simulate the perceived intentions of another is the basis of learning behaviours (Meltzoff et al., 2009) and our capacity to resonate with the internal state of another. However, this capacity to resonate is dependent on prior learning. As Daniel Siegel puts it:

If you are from New York City and I raise my hand in front of you, you may imagine that I am hailing a cab. If you are currently a student, you may imagine that I am intending to ask a question. If you have been abused, you may feel that I am going to hit you. Prior learning shapes the empathic interpretation and the internal simulation. (Siegel, 2012, p. 166)

This prior learning of the mirror-neuron system may have played a pivotal role "in our becoming the one and only species that veritably lives and breathes culture" (Ramachandran, 2011, p. 117)—a culture comprising an extraordinary complexity of knowledge, skills, and responses shared and passed down by way of language and imitation. Our unique ability to see the world from another's perspective and to construct mental models of another's thoughts and intentions (known as "theory of mind"), integral to the formation and transfer of culture, appears to rest—at least in part—on the capacity of our mirror-neuron system.

Looking at facial expressions is an activity that stimulates mirror neurons as we simulate the perceived expressions (Lundqvist & Dimberg, 1995), and this in turn activates the neural networks related to our own experience when we make those expressions. We see someone with a big, infectious smile, and we start to smile ourselves, even if it is very subtle. The inner experience we have lets us know what the smiling person must be experiencing.

If mirror neurons help us attune to others and develop empathy, then how should we understand the case of an autistic person, where there is a distinct lack of social intuition? It seems that the autistic have an impaired mirror-neuron system, leaving them with a limited capacity to learn through observation, emotionally attune, and behave empathically (Dapretto et al., 2006; Perkins, Stokes, McGillivray, & Bittar, 2010). While clearly there are additional factors involved in autism, this appears to be a crucial deficit. A series of studies by Ramachandran and colleagues used EEG to measure mirror-neuron activity via the suppression of mu-wave activity in autistic children. The subjects were found to produce mu-wave activity as normal children do, which was suppressed when they were asked to perform simple voluntary movements, as is healthy. However, when watching someone else perform an action that would normally suppress mu-wave activity (indicating mirror-neuron activity), the usual suppression did not occur (Ramachandran, 2011). Further independent studies have suggested that there is a reduced functional connection between the visual cortex and the prefrontal mirror-neuron system in autistic subjects.

Often autistic people will have difficulty with metaphorical language and take metaphors too literally. Ramachandran contends that this can be explained from the perspective of embodied cognition and a lack of mirror-neuron involvement in understanding metaphor. He and his colleagues noticed that patients with lesions in the left supramarginal gyrus who had apraxia also had difficulty with action-based metaphors like "Get a grip on yourself." The supramarginal gyrus contains mirror neurons, and the evidence suggests that a deficit of functional connectivity to this region can make it hard to interpret action-based metaphors.

Are these disconnects within the mirror-neuron system of autistics permanent? Keysers and colleagues performed experiments focusing on the facial expressions of higher-functioning autistic adults. They found that the activity in the mirror system of the youngest participants (aged around 18 years) was significantly low, as expected. But as age increased, the functionality of the insula and motor regions also steadily increased, until about the age of 30, when it was considered normal (Keysers, 2011). It seems the mirror system may not be broken, but delayed or hindered in making functional connections. This suggests that, at least in respect to the mirror system, the higher-functioning autistic brain does have mechanisms and a pathway to improved social integration and intuition.

Mirror neurons apparently play a role in our empathic attunement to others' experience of physical pain. The anterior cingulate is one area known to respond to physical pain, and it is this region that has been monitored during neurosurgery and in non-invasive neuroimaging studies. Monitoring sensory pain neurons that respond to pain receptors on the skin, researchers have found that these pain neurons also respond when the conscious patient sees another patient being poked, for example. Similar neurons for touch have been identified in the parietal lobe using brain-imaging techniques (Keysers, 2011).

The discovery of mirror neurons has enabled us to refine our model of the social brain. Although some researchers were guilty initially of overenthusiasm about mirror neurons and the role they might play in social perception, we have seen the pendulum swing back to a more sensible and integrative understanding of this system, as one of many that constitute our social brain. Mirror neurons are not the be-all and end-all of empathy and learning—they are but a part of a very complex interconnected whole. As with so many aspects of the brain, it is important to remember that it is not so much the individual functionality of mirror neurons that matters as the functional connectivity of the entire mirror-neuron system.

Some Key Areas of the Empathic Brain

(Cozolino, 2014; Keysers, 2011; Ramachandran, 2011)

- **Anterior cingulate cortex:**
  Links emotions and actions.

- **Inferior frontal gyrus:**
  Programs complex actions and language.

- **Insula:**
  Senses the inner state of the body and controls visceral responses, emotions.

- **Primary motor cortex:**
  Controls muscles.

- **Medial prefrontal cortex**:
  Performs cognitive processing of the states of the self and of others.

- **Premotor cortex:**
  Plans actions.

- **Parietal lobe:**
  Integrates information from all senses and programs responsive actions. An important synergy exists between the mPFC and parietal lobes to integrate space–time context with action plans/goals/relationships. Includes the supramarginal gyrus.

- **Primary & secondary somatosensory cortex:**
  Senses touch and the position of own body (proprioception).

- **Supplementary motor area:**
  Plans and controls actions.

- **Primary visual cortex:**
  Detects simple features in the visual information from the retina.

- **Temporal visual cortex:**
  Combines simple visual features detected by the primary visual cortex and sometimes information from auditory cortices into neurons responding to the perception of socially relevant entities (faces, actions, etc.).

DEFAULT MODE

THE PSYCHOTHERAPIST'S ESSENTIAL GUIDE TO THE BRAIN

We are social beings with sophisticated and complex systems of relating to one another. The psychological needs of pain avoidance, orientation/control, and attachment are very often social in nature: the satisfaction, violation, or deprivation of these needs happens primarily in a social context, impacting our self-esteem and sense of well-being. We feel real pain when betrayed by a friend, disorientation when we get mixed messages about our role at work, a breach of attachment when our spouse fails to let us know they are going to be late home. All our fundamental psychological needs are most fully satisfied or most severely violated in the social context.

In 1997, Gordon Shulman and colleagues (Shulman et al., 1997; Shulman, Fiez, et al., 1997) reanalysed nine previous positron emission tomography (PET) studies on visual processing to find out which brain regions were commonly activated across a diverse number of cognitive tasks: the first paper looked at common activation of regions when doing a task, and the second paper focused on common activation of regions when not doing a task. They made the surprising discovery that a shared set of brain regions was activated whenever subjects were resting from a cognitive task. These regions were initially given the label "task-induced deactivation network", and later renamed the default mode, or default mode network (DMN; Lieberman, 2013). Since these early studies, investigations using similar imaging-based techniques have continued, as researchers try to understand what the default network is doing and why.

The activation patterns of the DMN revolve around episodic memory, self-projection, and self-referential processing, located in hubs in both the medial prefrontal cortex (mPFC) and the posterior cingulate cortex (PCC). Centres include the precuneus, the orbital frontal gyrus, the anterior cingulate gyrus, the inferolateral temporal cortex, the parahippocampal gyrus, and the lateral parietal cortex (Buckner & Carroll, 2007; Fox et al., 2005; Konishi, McLaren, Engen, & Smallwood, 2015; Shulman et al., 1997; Thomason et al., 2008). In a nutshell, these activation patterns revolve around thoughts about ourselves and others and the relationships we have with others, remembering the past, and planning the future. Together they represent an automatic activation pattern that is always on when we are not focused on the external environment or on any particular cognitive task. We might be indulging in self-reflection, thinking about what others are thinking (theory of mind), re-evaluating a past conversation, or rehearsing a future one. The DMN network pattern that supports social thinking is deactivated when we engage in non-social thinking, and when we have finished with a non-social cognitive task the DMN immediately lights up again. This does not mean that the PFC does not light up with various individual nodes of the DMN during a non-social task, but rather that the broad DMN signature is not maintained during non-social cognition.

Recent studies have suggested that the DMN plays a role in higher-order cognition, allowing cognition to be shaped by information from stored representations (memory) as well as by information in the immediate environment (Konishi et al., 2015). According to Konishi and colleagues, the DMN may not be merely a "task-negative" system that is on when cognitive work stops, or a network that is only activated by social themes; rather, the main mPFC–PCC hubs of the DMN may allow cognition to be guided by memory instead of relying solely on immediate perceptual input (Konishi et al., 2015). Higher-order thinking that involves imagining the future, taking the perspective of another person, or other complex introspection relies on representations (memory) not present in the immediate external environment, and thus the DMN comes into play.

Matthew Lieberman, a specialist in social cognitive neuroscience, introduced a number of interesting shifts in perspective concerning the DMN (Lieberman, 2013). One of the most interesting was that we are primed to be so social *because* of this default activity, rather than the reverse: that we are socially interested and therefore default to this network. When we are at rest from specific cognitive tasks, it seems the brain is engaged with thoughts about the very complex social world. Perhaps, as Lieberman suggests, this is an important priming of our thought processes that enables us to be more socially savvy when we engage with others.

If we are so socially focused, and our default state is to be thinking about self, others, and relationships, then the question arises: Do individuals with autism spectrum disorder (ASD) have the same default mode? Not surprisingly, there seems to be a deficit in the connectivity of the DMN in those with ASD—and the stronger

Sagittal MRI slice with the precuneus shown in red.
Image: Geoff B. Hall - <u>Wikimedia Commons</u>

the symptoms, the greater the disconnect. Specifically, there is a lack of connective strength between the mPFC and the PCC (known as the default mode midline core) in those with ASD compared to control subjects, and the deficit increases with the severity of the autism (Yerys et al., 2015). ASD is commonly understood to be characterized by a hypo-connectivity between remote cortical regions and a hyper-connectivity within certain cortical regions—fewer global connections but more local connections, in other words. Along these lines, studies have found that children with ASD show a reduced connectivity between the regions that make up the DMN, and increased local connectivity within these same regions (Washington et al., 2013). The long-distance connections between regions increase during childhood development, peaking at around 11–13 years, but children with ASD fail to undergo the typical strengthening of connectivity within the DMN network in adolescence (Washington et al., 2013). Without normal DMN activation when at rest, the individual with ASD is not being primed—neither rehearsing nor evaluating their social situation, but rather defaulting to more specific processing within regions in a more neurally isolated way.

Increased functional connectivity within the DMN in conjunction with reduced connectivity between the DMN and the central executive network (CEN) has been correlated with major depressive disorder (MDD) (Ho et al., 2015; Posner et al., 2016)—a finding that makes intuitive sense given the depressed individual's immersive negative ruminations about self, others, past, future, and relationships. Depression may also involve a greater functional connectivity between the subgenual prefrontal cortex, which is associated with affect-heavy behavioural withdrawal, and the self-referential process of the DMN (Hamilton, Farmer, Fogelman, & Gotlib, 2015).

A recent study of interest suggests that the importance of religion or spirituality to a person can mitigate some of this increased DMN connectivity (Svob, Wang, Weissman, Wickramaratne, & Posner et al, 2016). The authors of this study found that individuals who were at high risk for MDD, and who also reported that religion/spirituality was very important to them, showed lower DMN connectivity than those high-risk participants who did not rate religion/spirituality as important. The importance of spirituality to an individual at risk of familial depression may support neural adaptation in the DMN in a protective manner. Unlike some previous research that found meditation-based activity reduced internal DMN connectivity and increased DMN-CEN connectivity, this study only found differences in the internal DMN connectivity, suggesting belief in religion/spirituality provides a different protective factor than that of the contemplative practices of mindfulness. Such a study does not determine whether the "chicken" came before the "egg", however: Does spirituality prevent the

Magnetic resonance imaging of areas of the brain in the default mode network. Image: John Graner, Neuroimaging Department, National Intrepid Center of Excellence, Walter Reed National Military Medical Center, MD, USA. Wikimedia Commons

This image shows main regions of the default mode network (in yellow) and connectivity between the regions colour-coded by structural traversing direction (xyz -> rgb).
Image: Andreas Horn. Wikimedia Commons

development of an overly connected DMN, or does the attenuation of such functional connectivity lend itself to spirituality?

There is evidence that exposure to trauma can disrupt the DMN in a somewhat different way to depression, although the exact relationship between trauma and the DMN remains unclear. One recent study has looked at veterans with PTSD, combat-exposed veterans, and never-traumatized civilian controls to see if trauma exposure, rather than a distinctly PTSD mechanism, can disrupt the DMN (DiGangi et al., 2016). The researchers found that there was a reduced DMN connectivity with the traumatized veterans—both the PTSD group and the non-PTSD yet combat-exposed veterans. The trauma-exposed veterans showed less precuneus to mPFC and right superior parietal lobule connectivity, regardless of PTSD diagnosis, suggesting it is the experience of combat trauma that that correlates with DMN changes. Similar DMN disruptions have been noted in other types of civilian trauma.

Altogether this is fascinating work, revealing the nature of our brains' default activity and highlighting the importance of the social fabric we navigate daily. So next time you find yourself mentally wandering off into a world of relationships, past conversations, and ruminations about yourself, you know your DMN is fully engaged.

A recent research study is paving the way for a non-invasive way to stimulate the vagus nerve to modulate the DMN and ward off depression (Fang et al., 2016). Vagus nerve stimulation is a somatic treatment for depression that has shown promise but traditionally involves surgery and can have significant side effects. The procedure involves a pacemaker-like device being surgically implanted in the body and attached to a stimulating wire connected to the vagus nerve. Now a Chinese-funded project is testing a non-invasive way of stimulating the vagus nerve, using a technique known as transcutaneous vagus nerve stimulation (tVNS), and modulating the functional connectivity of the DMN to improve depressive symptoms. The tVNS method capitalizes on the fact that the ear is probably the only place on the surface of the body where there is afferent vagus nerve distribution. Direct stimulation of the afferent nerve fibres on the ear is achieved by an electrode device that touches the auricular concha area of the outer ear where there are rich vagus-nerve branch distributions. The electrodes stimulate the vagus nerve to produce an effect similar to the traditional VNS procedure minus the complications of a surgical implant. Treatments were over a period of four weeks, with two 30-minute sessions daily at least five days a week. The research found that tVNS significantly reduced the severity of depression in subjects and produced significant changes in DMN brain regions involved in emotional modulation.

OBSESSIVE-COMPULSIVE

Obsessive–compulsive disorder (OCD) is a common anxiety condition characterized by recurring upsetting thoughts (obsessions), typically along the lines of contamination, doubts, the need to order things, impending doom, or aggression—to name just a few. These obsessions are managed by ritualistic actions (compulsions) such as hand washing, checking, ordering, counting, praying, and other sequences of action or thought. People who suffer from OCD feel driven to outwork specific compulsions to mitigate the anxiety generated by the obsessive thoughts. One of the more common OCD experiences is that of feeling contaminated and being compelled to wash the hands or the entire body to be clean again. The feeling of being clean either never happens or is fleeting, despite excessive efforts to wash. Another typical example is persistent doubt upon leaving the house that the house is locked and windows closed or that the oven has been turned off, and such persistent thoughts lead to compulsive checking—a distressing state that intrudes on the harmonious flow of life and torments the sufferer when they are not in a position to do the checking.

DSM-5 Diagnostic Criteria for Obsessive-Compulsive Disorder

American Psychiatric Association. (2013). *Diagnostic and statistical manual of mental disorders* (5th ed.). Washington, DC: American Psychiatric Publishing

A. Presence of obsessions, compulsions, or both:

Obsessions are defined by (1) and (2):

1. Recurrent and persistent thoughts, urges, or impulses that are experienced, at some time during the disturbance, as intrusive and unwanted, and that in most individuals cause marked anxiety or distress.

2. The individual attempts to ignore or suppress such thoughts, urges, or images, or to neutralize them with some other thought or action (i.e., by performing a compulsion).

Compulsions are defined by (1) and (2):

1. Repetitive behaviours (e.g., hand washing, ordering, checking) or mental acts (e.g., praying, counting, repeating words silently) that the individual feels driven to perform in response to an obsession or according to rules that must be applied rigidly.

2. The behaviours or mental acts are aimed at preventing or reducing anxiety or distress, or preventing some dreaded event or situation; however, these behaviours or mental acts are not connected in a realistic way with what they are designed to neutralize or prevent, or are clearly excessive.

B. The obsessions or compulsions are time-consuming (e.g., take more than 1 hour per day) or cause clinically significant distress or impairment in social, occupational, or other important areas of functioning.

C. The obsessive-compulsive symptoms are not attributable to the physiological effects of a substance (e.g., a drug of abuse, a medication) or another medical condition.

D. The disturbance is not better explained by the symptoms of another mental disorder (e.g., excessive worries, as in generalized anxiety disorder; preoccupation with appearance, as in body dysmorphic disorder; difficulty discarding or parting with possessions, as in hoarding disorder; hair pulling, as in trichotillomania [hair-pulling disorder]; skin picking, as in excoriation [skin-picking] disorder; stereotypies, as in stereotypic movement disorder; ritualized eating behaviour, as in eating disorders; preoccupation with substances or gambling, as in substance-related and addictive disorders; preoccupation with having an illness, as in illness anxiety disorder; sexual urges or fantasies, as in paraphilic disorders; impulses, as in disruptive, impulse-control, and conduct disorders; guilty ruminations, as in major depressive disorder; thought insertion or delusional preoccupations, as in schizophrenia spectrum and other psychotic disorders; or repetitive patterns of behaviour, as in autism spectrum disorder).

Neural Underpinnings of OCD

What is known about the neurobiological underpinnings of OCD? As brain-imaging technology becomes more sophisticated, we are starting to identify specific brain structures implicated in OCD and some of the neurochemicals involved in modulating the OCD response. Here we consider the circuits involved in OCD and the ramifications for treatment.

At a Parisian hospital in 1967, psychiatrist and neurosurgeon Jean Talairach and his team were investigating the origins of seizures in epileptic patients when they discovered that the stimulation of the cingulum resulted in compulsive behaviours. The cingulum, located directly above the corpus callosum in the cingulate gyrus, is involved in complex repetitive movements and has been implicated in a bigger circuit involved in OCD. This more elaborate neural circuit has become known as the OCD loop (Modell, Mountz, Curtis, & Greden, 1989) and includes the orbitofrontal cortex (OFC), striatum, and thalamus.

The OFC, covered in our earlier section on The Neocortex, is involved with the cognitive processing of decision making and expectation. It is an emotionally attuned part of the frontal cortex that is sensitive to threatening situations. Fed to the OFC is information from the striatum, a major part of the basal ganglia in-

A closer look at the loop

The OFC and anterior cingulate cortex (ACC) connect to the basal ganglia and the thalamus in what is known as the cortico–basal ganglia–**thalamocortical** (CBGTC) loop (Alexander, DeLong, & Strick, 1986). There are "direct" and "indirect" pathways through the basal ganglia that create an equilibrium of response to situations. This figure shows both pathways.

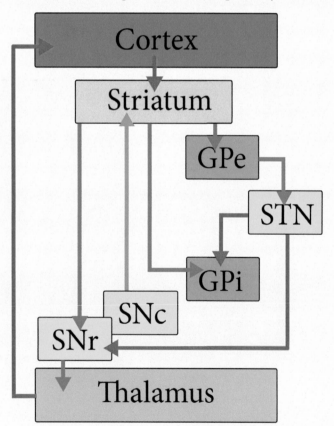

Direct pathways run from the cortex to the striatum, then to the globus pallidus internal segment (GPi) and substantia nigra pars reticulate (SNr), then to the thalamus, and finally back to the cortex. The glutamatergic pathways are in red, dopaminergic in magenta, and GABA in blue.

The indirect pathways run from the cortex to the striatum, then to the globus pallidus external segment (GPe), the subthalamic nucleus (STN), the GPi and SNr, then to the thalamus, and finally back to the cortex.

(Figure based on an image created by Andrew Gillies from Wikimedia Commons, https://commons.wikimedia.org/wiki/File%3ABasal-ganglia-classic.png)

The direct pathway is an excitatory one, whereas the indirect pathway is inhibitory. So it may be that relatively excessive activity in the direct pathway in these loops could result in positive feedback loops leading to OCD (Saxena & Rauch, 2000).

volved in reward and habit formation. It is the striatum that allows us to multitask by running automatic behaviour in the background, like the student who plays with her hair while listening to a challenging lecture. Part of the striatum, the caudate nucleus, working with the putamen, acts rather like an entrance or gate within the basal ganglia to activate or attenuate automatic responses. Part of what is believed to be happening in OCD is that when the striatum is not doing its gatekeeping job properly (i.e., the "entrance" is left open and unmanaged), obsessive thoughts and compulsions can flood the OFC uninhibited. There may be a "warning" from the amygdala about germs, for example, that prompts thoughts of washing hands. The OFC responds to such incoming information by reinforcing compulsive behaviours (such as hand washing) to "make things right". But a single action fails to satisfy the OFC, because there is an open loop in operation that recycles the "warning" signal (e.g., that there is still contamination) to the OFC. This hyperactivity of the OFC and the lack of inhibition by the dorsolateral prefrontal cortex (DLPFC) of the striatum could be one of the main causes of OCD.

The OFC receives messages from the amygdala that are sent back to the lateral amygdala. This fear circuit is mediated by the HPA axis (discussed in The Hypothalamus in our section on Deep Systems), and is further activated when sufferers of OCD do not engage in the compulsive behaviour—in other words, when they consciously stop the compulsive behaviour but the obsessive thoughts are still feeding back to the amygdala, letting the system know that "things are still not OK". With engagement in the compulsive behaviour there comes a temporary measure of relief, as the fear circuits are down-regulated. This management of fear and anxiety can lead to even more obsessive thinking and compulsive behaviours to avoid the uncomfortable consequences of an anxiety response.

Normally there is a balance between the OFC, the basal ganglia, and the thalamus that gives us flexibility as we activate or inhibit, in a situationally appropriate way, responses to thoughts and the environment. When the balance breaks down and there is less inhibition, as in the case of Tourette's syndrome, automatic behaviours become very difficult to inhibit. An OFC flooded with input from the basal ganglia needs help in inhibiting the automatic behaviour that is trying to "make things right". This help can come from the DLPFC—the part of the frontal cortex involved in positive, goal-orientated, reflective, and rational behaviour—which can assist the more emotionally driven OFC in putting the brakes on the obsessive–compulsive loop. This is achieved by strengthening the control the OFC has over the amygdala to shut down the fear network. The DLPFC can strengthen attentional skills (such as focusing on the present moment, reframing, tolerance, and acceptance) and override the automatic and habitual flow from the OFC, in effect distracting the OFC from autopilot and training it to engage in something more beneficial than the habitual OCD response. As clients in therapy learn to ignore the compulsive urges and see the behaviour as non-functional, they can establish stronger connections from the OFC to the amygdala and regain control over what was an uninhibited autopilot of fear.

Some theory postulates a delayed maturation of the frontal cortex–striatum circuitry, where the maturation of the cingulate is a causal factor in OCD (Rosenberg & Keshavan, 1998). Neuroimaging studies have shown higher activity in the OFC, ACC, and striatum in OCD patients than non-OCD subjects.

Neurochemistry of OCD

The nucleus accumbens, also referred to as the "pleasure centre" of the brain, is a region in the basal forebrain shown in the diagram below. This area, rich in dopaminergic neurons, plays a central role in reward behaviour. Engaging in OCD behaviour to down-regulate the stress response and resolve internal anxiety is also inherently rewarding, as it increases the dopaminergic activity in the brain. Other neurotransmitter activity that seems to be important in the OCD loop is that of glutamate and GABA between the OFC and caudate nucleus, the globus pallidus, and the thalamus. Dopamine modulates the activity of the caudate nucleus, and serotonin modulates the activity of the globus pallidus. Although OCD patients do not typically show serotonin deficits, when they are placed on serotonin reuptake inhibitors (SRIs), 40–60% show improvements of symptoms. Similarly, administering a dopamine antagonist can be effective in reducing motor tics, indicating dopamine as a possible modulator of behavioural compulsions in OCD.

Psychopharmacological therapy today revolves around the use of SRIs/SSRIs, even though there is not a good explanation as to why increasing serotonin levels improves OCD symptoms. Clomipramine (Anafranil) was the first SRI demonstrated to bring improvement in some cases of OCD. It blocks 5-HT (serotonin) and norepinephrine uptake and has some dopamine receptor-blocking function. This class of SRI has more side effects than more recent SSRIs such as fluoxetine (Prozac), sertraline (Zoloft), paroxetine (Paxil), and fluvoxamine (Luvox). Sometimes anxiolytics like benzodiazepines are used at the same time to combat the anxiety associated with OCD. It is difficult to judge how effective these pharmacological therapies are, and most approaches are a combination of chemical intervention and some form of cognitive behavioural therapy.

nucleus accumbens

Therapeutic Intervention

As stated above, the DLPFC is the brain region that can be utilized to break the OCD loop by reorientation of the OFC away from its obsessive–compulsive drive. By activating the DLPFC (in conjunction with the hippocampus) to take executive control over thoughts and behaviour, recognizing that OCD behaviour is not adaptive, and laying down new neural traces that are more adaptive, the OFC can be retrained. The most common approach to this is through CBT techniques such as exposure and response prevention (ERP), first developed in the 1970s. By exposing clients gradually and systematically, with careful

Coronal slices of human brain showing the basal ganglia. White matter is shown in dark grey, grey matter is shown in light grey. Anterior: striatum, globus pallidus (GPe and GPi) Posterior: subthalamic nucleus (STN), substantia nigra (SN). Image by Andrew Gillies - https://commons.wikimedia.org/wiki/File:Basal-ganglia-coronal-sections-large.png

cognitive processing, the abnormal portico-ganglia circuit can be rewired to function in a much more adaptable and flexible way. Research has indicated that OCD patients who engage in such CBT therapy do have decreased metabolism in the right caudate nucleus in the basal ganglia, a decrease in thalamus activity, and an increase in right-side ACC activity (Linden, 2006; Saxena et al., 2009). A practical and up-to-date workbook for clients is *Brain Based Therapy for OCD: A Workbook for Clinicians and Clients*, by John Arden.

FEAR & ANXIETY

In the previous section we examined the neural substrates of OCD. In this section we turn our attention to some of the neuroscience behind other anxiety disorders such as phobias, panic attacks, post-traumatic stress disorder (PTSD) and generalized anxiety disorder (GAD). These anxiety disorders can become debilitating, and as clinicians we encounter them often among the problems clients approach us for help with. We thus have a unique opportunity to learn the neural mechanisms involved in anxiety disorders and to evaluate interventions against a sound understanding of what is taking place in a client's nervous system. Here we begin with the neurological bases of fear and anxiety, and continue in more detail in the second half of this section.

The emotional response of fear and anxiety is, of course, adaptive. It is a natural response designed to keep us safe from a perceived threat, be it physical or a more complex social/emotional threat. On one level we can appreciate that apprehension about failing an exam can motivate us to study a little harder, or that fear of losing our job spurs us to get to work on time. But when these adaptive and useful mechanisms become exaggerated and go into "overdrive", we have a problem: rather than achieving the goal of keeping us safe, fear cripples us, robbing us of a normal life. So what constitutes our fear mechanism, how does it become maladaptive, and what can we do about it?

The Rats of Fear

Joseph LeDoux has devoted his career to mapping out the fear network of the brain. By conditioning rats to elicit a fear response associated with a certain stimulus (a tone), LeDoux was able to trace the neural pathways of fear. His early experiments involved lesioning the auditory cortex to prevent the rats from "hearing" the feared stimuli, the assumption being that without auditory processing the rats would not respond with fear. Surprisingly, the rats continued to respond to the tone with fear after the lesion. How could the animals know to fear the tone without being able to process it in their auditory cortex? The fear network was unaffected, meaning that its mechanism must be operational before auditory information reaches the auditory cortex; that is, there must be a pathway other than that of the thalamus–cortex. And it happens that there is. LeDoux developed the neuroscience of fear based on a non-cortical pathway he called the "low road"—a fast, direct pathway that requires no higher-order thought to activate a physiological response to a threat.

LeDoux's rats, which had learned to fear a specific tone, processed incoming auditory information from the thalamus directly to the amygdala—the small, almond-shaped fear-learning centre that was covered in our section on Deep Systems. LeDoux demonstrated the important role the amygdala plays in learning and memory. He showed that the auditory information entering the amygdala, specifically the basal and lateral aspects (known as the basolateral complex of the amygdala or BLA), has not been analysed by higher cortical processing, and that seemingly any tone that is similar to the conditioned tone will trigger a warning from the amygdala. In fact, all sensory information from the thalamus arrives first at the amygdala—the fast "low road" of information processing. The "high road" is a slower pathway that facilitates the passage of sensory information through the cortex before meeting the "low road" back at the amygdala. This slower pathway adds much more detail and character to the raw data as it is analysed in "smarter" parts of the brain. To illustrate, after an immediate and instinctive jump at a snake-like object on the ground, our "high road" processing recognizes the object as a hose rather than a snake, and this discrimination down-regulates the fear response. The output of the amygdala is connected to many neural structures that activate either the freeze response or the fight-or-flight response together with other systems to raise arousal levels and direct attention. It is the fast, unconscious "low road" of information processing that may be responsible for initiating panic attacks that appear to come out of nowhere. As an oversensitive amygdala springs into action, it instantly draws oxygen-rich blood flow from areas such as the right orbitofrontal cortex and anterior cingulate cortex (important for modulating the response of the amygdala), leaving the sufferer with that out-of-control feeling of dread and/or panic as a cascade of stress chemicals activates their body to deal with imminent danger.

The implicit emotional learning of the amygdala is unlike the explicit memory of places, events, and facts that is mediated by the hippocampus. The explicit learning of the contextual details of a fear-related incident is hippocampal-dependent. The memories of context by themselves are not emotional; emotional aspects of memory require amygdala activity and the pairing of contextual elements with the emotional representation of those elements. Unlike the rats in LeDoux's lab, we can make emotional associations just by recognizing a dangerous situation from context, with our amygdala coming into play to encode an emotional element to the learning—a helpful skill to have when the feared stimuli are oncoming trucks, exposed power lines, guns, or strange men offering a ride.

Fear vs. Anxiety

Fear is a response to a specific stimulus while that stimulus poses a threat. It is fear that motivates us to move out of the way of an oncoming vehicle, but once the vehicle has passed, it no longer poses a threat. Anxiety, however, is a different matter—it does not necessarily require a trigger, but is the anticipation of a threat. Anxiety is the continual vigilance for potential threats, an energy-consuming alertness for danger even if there is no immediate danger. In the consistency model of mental functioning described by Klaus Grawe, this state is characterized by an active avoidance network that is always scanning for potential threats, never quite satisfied that all is safe (Grawe, 2007). It arises through a combination of an oversensitive amygdala and a reduction in the capacity of other brain regions to modulate

the amygdala response. In some cases, the vigilance for threats can be generalized into what is known as generalized anxiety disorder (GAD), where the sufferer demonstrates a hypervigilance for threat and avoidance of anything that could be threatening but in a very diffuse, rather indiscriminate manner. For this individual, much of the environment—people, places, things—feels like a potential threat and either must be avoided or at best evokes a sense of unease.

Extinction

We have learned from LeDoux's work with rats that a fear memory can be created by pairing a shock with a tone, so that eventually the tone by itself will elicit fear. One of the key concepts that follows from this process of fear memory creation is that of "extinction": the unlearning of fear. If the tone that was previously associated with a shock is repeatedly sounded without any shock, a new learning is created, and the tone is eventually associated with no shock. This is the basis of exposure therapy. It is not *forgetting*, but rather a new memory association. Indeed, "extinction" may be a misnomer, as what is happening seems more like the creation of yet another neural network of association that competes with the previous learning. It has been observed that in different contexts or under stress the old learning (tone = shock) can rear its head again despite attempts at extinction.

The ventral medial prefrontal cortex (vmPFC),

which was introduced earlier in this series, is integral to our "emotional brain" and has direct bilateral connections with the amygdala. The vmPFC can regulate the emotional response of the amygdala by "updating" the amygdala's "firmware" as new information becomes available. The thickness of the vmPFC is positively correlated with ease in acquiring an extinction memory in the normal population. Another brain region associated with fear expression is the dorsal aspect of the anterior cingulate cortex (dACC). It has been hypothesized that sufferers of PTSD have a problem recalling the newer extinction memory (e.g., a walk down the street where snipers were *not* shooting at you), so that the earlier fear conditioning remains dominant. An increase in vmPFC and hippocampal activity has been positively correlated with extinction recall, whereas increased dACC activity (the dACC has excitatory connections with the amygdala) is correlated with fear expression. In normal circumstances, the vmPFC, orbitofrontal cortex, and anterior cingulate cortex play a collaborative and integrative role with the amygdala in regulating physiological/emotional responses to danger. Some studies have observed that PTSD patients show a joint decrease in vmPFC and left anterior cingulate activity and increased right amygdala activity in response to a fear stimulus. Decreased volume and activation of the hippocampus has also been implicated in PTSD, which may account for a disturbed encoding of the traumatic event at the time it happened and the reintegration of that information upon recall. The overall picture is that of an under-regulated, hypersensitive amygdala with poor integration across various key neural circuits that would normally put implicit emotional memory within an appropriate context.

Both fear learning and extinction learning are, in reality, a complexity of interactions among brain regions such as those we have touched on above, facilitated by a neural plasticity that is dependent on brain-derived neurotrophic factor (BDNF) and N-methyl D-aspartate (NMDA) glutamate receptors. This complexity has given rise to difficulties such as that the use of selective serotonin reuptake inhibitors (SSRIs) reduces the

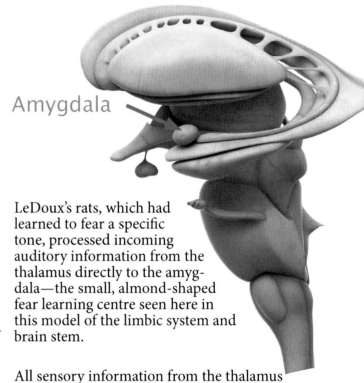

Amygdala

LeDoux's rats, which had learned to fear a specific tone, processed incoming auditory information from the thalamus directly to the amygdala—the small, almond-shaped fear learning centre seen here in this model of the limbic system and brain stem.

All sensory information from the thalamus first arrives at the amygdala—the fast "low road" of information processing.

GAD Brain Circuits

Research suggests that GAD sufferers can have weaker white matter connections (high-speed myelinated neural connections) between emotion-regulating areas of the brain such as the PFC, ACC, and amygdala. A major highway of this interconnectivity is the uncinate fasciculus, which helps us differentiate situations that are truly concerning from those that are merely annoyances. Mixed-up wiring can occur between the basolateral amygdala and the ventromedial amygdala—both of which extend to various regions of the brain. In GAD these areas of the amygdala are not as well connected with their normal targets, but there is a greater connectivity with the executive control network (ECN), and hypo-connectivity within the ECN. Such connectivity problems can reduce the ability to correctly evaluate and tolerate uncertainty and ambiguity, disrupt the balance between top-down and bottom-up control processes, and increase anxiety.

The Vagal Nerve System

The vagus complex is a multi-branch system of nerves linking the brain to the body. Two main routes of the vagal system are the dorsal vagal complex and the ventral vagal complex. The dorsal route begins in the brain stem and goes down into the abdominal organs and the heart. The ventral route, which is faster than the dorsal route because it is myelinated, extends from the nucleus ambiguus into the organs of the thoracic cavity, including the heart. This ventral complex has been called the social engagement system because it connects the expression of lower facial muscles with the activity of the organs in the thorax. It is the vagal nervous system that balances the sympathetic and parasympathetic branches of the autonomic nervous system, allowing us to calm down after an anxious response.

functionality of NMDA receptors that are required for successful extinction learning. Nevertheless, there are some promising findings in the realm of neurochemistry, such as chemical modulators that can enhance or suppress the synaptic plasticity that underlies fear or extinction learning. Ultimately, pharmacological treatments still have a long way to go.

Heart Rate Variability

A further aspect of fear and anxiety regulation involves the coordination between sympathetic and parasympathetic arousal measured by heart rate variability (HRV)—the subtle differences in timing between heart beats. A high HRV mediated through the vagus nerve and stellate ganglia indicates a healthy flexibility of attention to current situations, whereby healthy feedback mechanisms maintain an appropriate balance between the two branches of the autonomic nervous system (ANS) and thus a balanced response to various stimuli. The complexity of neural networks that maintains such regulation has been variously labelled the central autonomic network (CAN), the anterior executive region (AER), and the rostral limbic system. These descriptions attempt to capture the interplay between structures such as the ACC, insula, orbitofrontal cortex, amygdala, central grey, ventral striatum, brainstem, and ventral/dorsal vagal system, which perform a balancing act of the ANS. Some research has found that individuals with GAD have a reduced HRV because of a breakdown in the regulatory feedback mechanisms in the CAN resulting in chronic hyperarousal.

The Vagal Complex

Generally it can be said that all fear and anxiety disorders share the same hypersensitive amygdala response to a stimulus and disruption of regulatory circuits. The fear response engages the sympathetic nervous system (the fight-or-flight instinct) and disengages the ventral vagal branch of the parasympathetic system (the "social" system). However, if the perceived threat becomes overwhelming to the point of absolute terror, the sympathetic system can shut down and the dorsal vagal parasympathetic system activate, putting us into a dissociated *freeze* response. In this last-ditch effort to escape death by feigning death, the medial prefrontal cortex and anterior cingulate cortex shut down emotional arousal; the brainstem throws the body into shutdown (slowing the heart rate and metabolism and lowering blood pressure), and dissociation allows the sufferer mentally to go "elsewhere".

Approach & Avoid

So far, we have learned that the amygdala can act as an early-warning system for things that appear to be threatening, and that when the amygdala is triggered by an apparent threat, it starts a chain reaction of physiological responses to address the threat. First, corticotrophin-releasing hormone (CRH) signals the pituitary gland to release adrenocorticotrophic hormone (ACTH), which in turn signals the adrenal glands (situated above each kidney) to release adrenalin and then cortisol. This fear reaction takes place in what we call the hypothalamic–pituitary–adrenal (HPA) axis and is the best-known response to stress. But during a stress response the amygdala is simultaneously busy with other actions, such as signalling the locus coeruleus in the brainstem to release norepinephrine (NE), or noradrenaline. When the locus coeruleus is activated by stress, its increasing NE secretions alter prefrontal cognitive function, which has the knock-on effect of increasing motivation through the nucleus accumbens, increasing sympathetic and inhibiting parasympathetic tone as well as activating the HPA axis. Similarly, when NE is released by the locus coeruleus, there is greater activity in the right prefrontal cortex (R-PFC) and less activity in the left prefrontal cortex (L-PFC), hindering the latter's capacity to be verbally expressive in the face of growing anxiety. Excessive NE release can impair PFC function more generally and disinhibit the amygdala, leading to a state where the amygdala effectively "hijacks" the PFC. As a result, we are unable to rationalize the fear and anxiety we are feeling.

Experiencing fear and anxiety leads to the development of avoidant behaviour mediated by the R-PFC in order to avoid the triggering stimuli, whatever they may be. Continued avoidant behaviour has a rewarding effect (reinforced by dopamine), so that we become entrenched in the avoidance and end up enhancing and fortifying R-PFC activity at the expense of the more approach-oriented activity of the L-PFC. In effect, the more we avoid, and the more we allow the avoidant behaviour to develop, the harder it becomes to change. Teaching clients to "avoid" avoidant behaviour, therefore, lies at the heart of exposure therapy aimed at reversing the effects of chronic anxiety.

To increase activity in the L-PFC, it is vital to promote approach behaviours. This area of the brain is much better at processing details, maintaining positivity, and problem-solving than the R-PFC, which can get lost in the negative global "overwhelm" of irrational anxiety. In GAD, for example, there can be a gloomy, anxiety-provoking gestalt—when you can't quite put your finger on the exact problem—and it is at this moment that projections from the L-PFC, particularly the left medial PFC (lmPFC), can inhibit the activity of the amygdala and put the brakes, so to speak, on the habitual anxiety loop. By focusing on discrete details of specific behaviours, in incremental steps, we can walk clients through controllable incongruence toward greater L-PFC control. Controllable incongruence is a process of neural change in which the learning capacity of the brain is maximized by challenging what is habitual (e.g., R-PFC-mediated avoidant behaviour) in a way that feels controllable—albeit uncomfortable—and not overwhelming. It is important to regulate the process and get it "just right": insufficient challenge to the status quo will fail to stimulate new learning; too great a challenge will inhibit any new learning. Between these extremes lies the Goldilocks "just right" solution: a moderate increase in NE (challenge) and sustained beta endorphin activation to facilitate positive neural changes. In this way, graded exposure can rewire the brain.

When someone is challenged to face a fear in a way that enables them to feel in control (what is called "controllable incongruence"), moderate amounts of stress hormones such as cortisol and glutamate help them to stay alert, energized, and engaged so that new learning is facilitated through the optimization of neural plasticity. On the other hand, when the challenge—or stress—is escalated, and levels of norepinephrine, corticotrophin-releasing hormone (CRF) and cortisol rise, the amygdala is overactivated, and the conditions for new learning are degraded. High levels of stress hormones will break down the synaptic connections of new learning, and in an attempt to keep us safe, the brain will revert to the old avoidant networks. This is because elevated and chronic stress raises glutamate levels excessively and overactivates the NMDA receptors responsible for long-term potentiation of new learning, damaging what could have been a new neural pathway.

Aside from the R-PFC/L-PFC (avoid/approach) axis, another important consideration when dealing with anxiety disorders is the difference between bottom-up and top-down processing. The lmPFC regulation of amygdala activity is an example of top-down processing, and the combined amygdala and locus-coeruleus activation of the stress response is an example of bottom-up processing. Top-down processing is the slow-path, "high road" processing discussed earlier in this section, and bottom-up processing is the fast-track, "low road" response route that leads from the thalamus to the amygdala. Needless to say, clients in the grip of anxiety experience dominant bottom-up activation and are unable to access top-down processing in the form of PFC control over the amygdala. Top-down regulation of emotion involves dorsolateral and medial PFC and anterior cingulate cortex (ACC) control over limbic structures such as at the amygdala. When there is better top-down control, we can observe ventromedial and ventrolateral PFC activity to a greater depth in the cortex.

Bolstering Top-Down Processing

There are a number of strategies we can use with clients to bolster top-down processing, enhance approach-oriented thinking, and mitigate undue anxiety. But it is essential to start with a bottom-up approach: this means dealing with the strongest limbic-initiated physiological responses before attempting to address the higher cognitive processes. Clearly cognitive therapy is not going to be very effective while the client's PFC is "offline" and therefore unlikely to be very "cognitive". Somatically orientated therapeutic techniques can be especially effective to ground the client and calm an overactive amygdala.

Some form of focused breathing technique is a common and easy way to begin calming an anxious client. A mindful breathing exercise, for example, has multiple benefits. Activation of the parasympathetic nervous system during long, controlled outward breaths, which calms the nervous system and helps put the brakes on the HPA axis, is one important benefit; L-PFC activation while the client pays focused attention to the sensation of breathing, with a corresponding perfusion of the PFC as blood flows back to the frontal part of the brain from the deeper limbic regions, is another. This blood flow helps to prevent hyperventilation and retain the right amount of carbon dioxide (CO_2) in the bloodstream. Note that excessive exhalation of CO_2 will

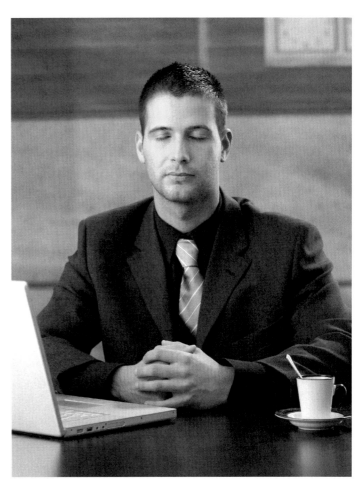

produce many of the physiological sensations associated with panic, due to the lowering of blood pH (hypocapnic alkalosis).

Other techniques such as a body scan or progressive muscle relaxation exercise, or indeed any mindfulness exercise (meditation, yoga, prayer), will activate the L-PFC as the client pays focused attention—whether on *interoceptive* (within the body) or *exteroceptive* (outside the body) stimuli. For example, noticing one's breathing, heartbeat, muscle tension and other feelings, and then wrapping language around the sensations that are the focus of that attention, will activate the left hemisphere. This activation can restrict the right hemisphere from dominating with the impression of being completely immersed in anxiety, and create some mental distance from the physiological symptoms. As a result, the observing self can emerge, and a greater sense of control can begin to develop.

As the client practises focused attention, or mindfulness, stronger and faster neural control networks will be built from the PFC to the limbic system. Mindful breathing and other mindfulness exercises can be established in a daily routine to strengthen PFC–limbic networks, restore balance through a healthier level of activation in the left hemisphere, and maintain frontal-lobe perfusion. With these bottom-up processes restored to a healthy level, the groundwork has been laid for effective work on top-down processes.

Cognitive approaches to anxiety address some of the errors in thought we are particularly prone to, such as polarization, catastrophizing, and automatic negative thoughts, all of which are associated with R-PFC-biased thinking. One of the keys to debunking cognitive misconceptions is to let your client know they need to give their PFC time to process what is happening rather than just go along with the amygdala's attempt to hijack the entire mental process. When negative or unhelpful automatic thoughts arise, they are more than likely a response to implicit memory activated by an overreactive amygdala. The client needs to take pause and think, "What is really going on here?" This gives the PFC time to become aware of the present moment, to appraise the current situation, and to decide on a more helpful, approach-oriented response as warranted by the current situation. Part of this approach orientation may take the

form of reframing assumptions in a graduated way. For example, a client may be anxious and becoming panicky about a social outing later in the week. Stopping and appraising what is really happening in the moment, and taking time to think, "I'm in my apartment, on a Tuesday night, watching TV" can allow a better perspective. It enables the client to recognize, "There is no immediate pressure to perform socially right now; I'm just watching TV alone, and this is relaxing," and provides an opportunity to reframe a negative assumption: "I'm learning to be more socially competent, and this Friday night I'll be better than the last time I went out." On the client's part, cultivating such approach-oriented cognitions—and following up by actually going out and not cancelling—provides the exposure (controllable incongruence) that can rewire the brain towards an L-PFC approach bias. Even just imagining doing OK and having positive social interactions at the next social event can begin to stimulate the client's social brain.

Narrative therapy can further reconstruct core beliefs about self (those beliefs that fuel negative, passive, global R-PFC thinking) in the form of more positive, active, detailed L-PFC appraisals of self and the world that can mitigate deep-seated anxiety. The core principles and techniques of acceptance and commitment therapy (ACT) also provide a complete suite of therapeutic interventions to cultivate "psychological flexibility"—again essentially a bolstering of L-PFC, top-down control. Generally speaking, the most effective techniques in this area aim to redress a bias in brain activity of the bottom-up, right-brained kind and restore a balance with top-down, left-brained processes.

On reading this brief review of "high road" and "low road" processing and the inherent tensions of the R-PFC/L-PFC (avoid/approach) axis to anxiety, the reader may be tempted to think of the R-PFC and bottom-up processes as the villain in this psychological drama. Don't be misled. The right hemisphere is imperative for a global perspective capable of tolerating the inevitable ambiguities of life, and bottom-up processes are vital to keeping us alive (see Iain McGilchrist's *The Master and His Emissary* for an expert and eye-opening exposition on the right hemisphere). But when normal flexible processing is hijacked by a hypersensitive alarm system, then restoring a healthy balance becomes a priority. As therapists, we can guide clients toward this goal by working to increase parasympathetic tone and by introducing graded exposure (controllable incongruence) in safe environments, thereby establishing better L-PFC control over reactions.

■ ■ ■ ■ ■ ■ ■ ■ ■ ■ ■ ■ ■ ■ ■ ■ ■ ■ ■

Increasing Parasympathetic Tone

Basic "bottom-up" techniques can be used with clients to increase their parasympathetic tone and put the brakes on a runaway anxiety response. For example:

- **Stop and breathe:** Controlled, focused breathing, especially a long, deep outward breath, activates the parasympathetic nervous system, slowing the heart rate and allowing blood to perfuse the PFC as the client maintains a point of focus (their breathing).

- **Relaxed posture:** Sitting, lying and/or stretching in a relaxed and mindful way (yoga is great for ideas here) can defuse bodily tensions.

- **Mindful attention:** A focus on the here and now, whether the focal point is within the body (*interoceptive*) or outside the body (*exteroceptive*), activates the L-PFC and down-regulates the amygdala.

- **Observing without judgement:** Observing bodily sensations without making any judgement about self or symptom can allow the "observing self" to emerge, affording a degree of detachment from the symptoms of anxiety. This (healthy) detachment from the symptoms and the self can be enhanced by labelling bodily sensations and thoughts: "I can feel my heart is racing" or "I'm having the thought that things will not be OK".

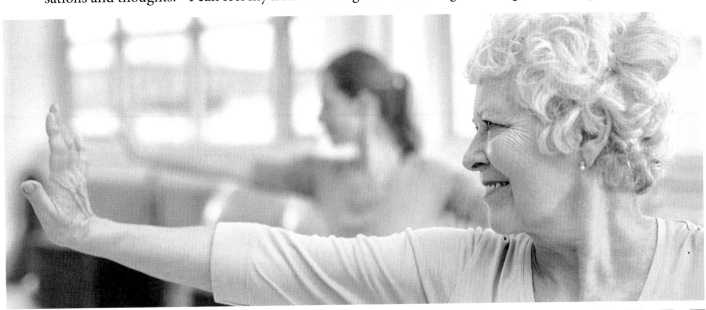

PAIN

Professor Matthew Lieberman heads the Social Cognitive Neuroscience Laboratory at UCLA and is the author of *Social: Why Our Brains Are Wired to Connect* (Lieberman, 2013). He and his colleagues have done important work in discovering the neural underpinnings of social pain and how it correlates with physical pain. All of us would recognize that the language we use to describe social pain employs the same words and phrases commonly used to describe physical pain: "She broke my heart," "I'm so cut up about it," "He really hurt me," "They stabbed me in the back!" and so on—and the phenomenon appears common across cultures and languages. There is a strong linguistic overlap between physical and social–emotional pain. But is there an actual neural overlap? This is the question that neuroscientists like Professor Lieberman have been investigating: Can the social pain of rejection, exclusion, or ostracism share the same or similar neural mechanisms as physical pain?

One of the regions of the brain under investigation is the dorsal anterior cingulate cortex (dACC). You may recall from our section on The Neocortex that the anterior cingulate cortex (ACC) is the front part of the cingulate cortex, commonly understood to be employed in error detection, with the dorsal (top) part associated with cognitive processing and the ventral (bottom) part with emotional processing. Studies have suggested that the dACC is involved in processing the distress of both physical and social pain—rather like an alarm system that both detects a problem and elicits a response. The dACC seems to monitor for discrepancies between one's goals and one's most habitual or predominant responses. When there is an inconsistency, the dACC lets the lateral prefrontal cortex know that it needs to intervene with a contextually appropriate response. The Stroop test is a good illustration, in that when subjects are shown colour words in odd colours (e.g., the word "red" written in blue) and asked to state the colour rather than the word, the dACC detects an inconsistency with the prepotent response to pronounce

the word rather than identify its colour (i.e., the correct answer for the word "red" written in blue is blue, but the tendency is to answer red). The dACC also functions to create attention-getting affective states such as pain, anxiety, and distress. Lieberman (2013) likens the ACC to an alarm system in that it can detect certain conditions (such as goal conflicts) and "sound the alarm".

As far back as the 1970s, the work of Jaak Panksepp and colleagues suggested that there was more than a metaphorical link between social and physical pain. These neuroscientists were looking at opiate receptor systems (the dACC is rich in receptors for endorphins, the brain's natural opioids) and found that both physical and social pain were modulated by such systems. Later studies found that even non-opioid pain relievers like Tylenol (acetaminophen) could ease social pain and that they reduced activity in the dACC (DeWall et al., 2010). The theory developed that since infant mammalian social needs are an issue of life or death—a baby mammal won't last long without social attachment—a system that monitors social–psychological proximity to caregivers is of vital importance. The idea was that a system that could detect an attachment breach and sound an alarm to elicit a reconnection would share some of the same neural processing as physical pain—

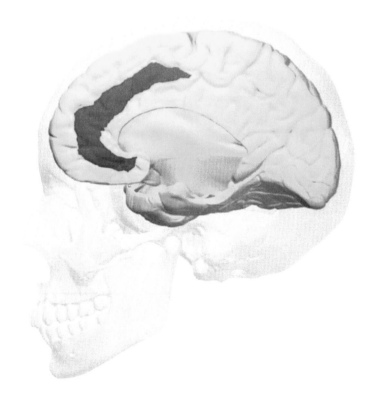

The dorsal anterior cingulate cortex is also know as Brodmann area 32 and plays a part in pain detection rather like an alarm system. 3D brain image from Anatomography another trigger for a survival response.

It is an enticing idea that the brain responds to social rejection using the same circuitry that encodes physical pain, but it is likely not this way on a neural level. In 2014, Choong-Wan Woo and colleagues at the University of Colorado, Boulder (Woo et al., 2014) found that the two kinds of pain are processed in the same areas but with different neural representations. In fact, they found that the encoding of physical pain and social rejection occurred in distinct global (whole-brain) patterns as well as different patterns within the pain-processing regions. So there may be a sharing of regions when processing the two types of pain, but research suggests there are distinct neural representations for each (see also Iannetti, Salomons, Moayedi, Mouraux, & Davis, 2013).

The system of the brain involved in the perception of and response to physical pain is known as the pain matrix. It comprises the dACC, rostral (front) ACC (rACC), somatosensory cortex, insula, periaqueductal grey, and right ventral prefrontal cortex (RVPFC). The insula and somatosensory cortex are primarily concerned with the sensory aspect of pain, while the periaqueductal grey, rACC, and RVPFC are more concerned with the regulation of pain through the release of opioids and cognitive processing. The dACC seems to be involved more in the subjective aspect of distress. There is a high correlation between the sensory intensity and subjective distress of pain, but the two can be separated. In the 1960s, chronic pain sufferers would sometimes elect to have a cingulotomy (a lesioning of the anterior cingulate) that would significantly decrease the subjective aspect of pain, although the sensory aspect continued—they could feel the pain, but it didn't bother them. By contrast, in cases where the somatosensory cortex is damaged, they experience distress from pain but have difficulty perceiving where the pain is coming from. It seems sensory intensity and subjective distress are two different neural circuits.

In a fascinating study on social exclusion, Matthew Lieberman, Naomi Eisenberg, and Kipling Williams performed a neuroimaging experiment on subjects to see what regions would be activated during social rejection (Eisenberger, Lieberman, & Williams, 2003). The subjects were placed in an fMRI scanner and told they would be playing a ball-tossing computer game with others who were also in scanners, in order to work out the technical details of a new neuroimaging procedure called hyperscanning. In fact there were no other subjects in scanners, only a computer posing as the other subjects. During the first scan, the subject was told that there was a technical problem and that he or she could watch the other two players toss the ball between themselves but would not be able to join them. In the second scan, the subject was able to join in the game and was fully included, with a 50% probability of being

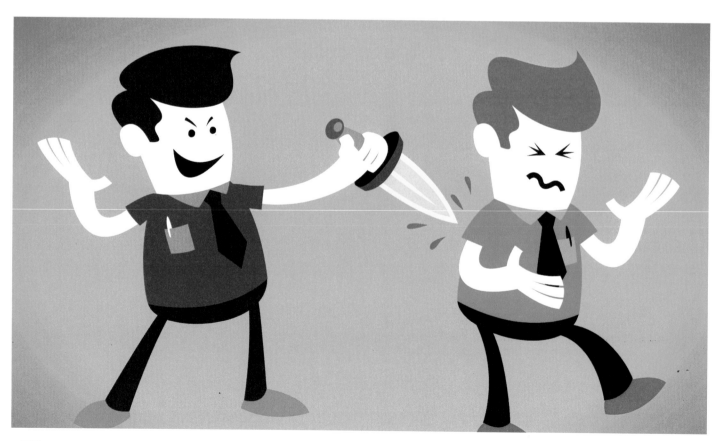

thrown the ball. In the final scan, the subject was initially included but after about 30 seconds was excluded from the ball throwing for the rest of the session—the appearance was that the other two "players" were having more fun tossing the ball to each other than including the (real) subject. After the scans, each subject filled out a questionnaire assessing the amount of social pain they experienced during the last scan.

During the exclusion trial, greater dACC, right insula, and RVPFC activity was observed than in the second scan when the subject was included in the ball tossing. There appeared to be a strong correlation between activity in the dACC and RVPFC and social pain. The pattern is similar to that in studies of physical pain, which have shown increased dACC, insula, and RVPFC activity. Further outcomes of such studies have indicated that the dACC mediates the relationship between self-reports of pain and RVPFC activity, substantiating the idea that the dACC produces the subjective level of distress but it is the RVPFC that intervenes to down-regulate the experience of such pain. Interestingly, the researchers found that dACC activity was also elevated when the subject was told there was a technical fault and they were excluded from the game. Is it possible that we are sufficiently hardwired in our response to social exclusion that the mere suggestion of it will provoke an automatic response in our dACC "alarm system"? In this scenario, however, there was no increase in RVPFC activity, presumably because the subjects had no reason to think they were being deliberately excluded.

If social and physical pain do indeed share neural substrates, what does that mean for us? Naomi Eisenberger looked into the consequences of such an overlap when she examined the possibility that an individual's sensitivity to physical pain positively correlated with their sensitivity to social pain (Eisenberger, 2012). She discovered a significant correlation, showing that a greater sensitivity to physical pain went hand-in-hand with greater pain upon social rejection. Earlier findings reviewed by Eisenberger showed that subjects with a variability in the μ-opioid receptor gene OPRM1 (carrying the G allele), which is associated with greater sensitivity to physical pain, also demonstrated greater sensitivity to social pain. Researchers had also tested to see if one sort of pain modulated the other, finding that physical pain tended to increase the sense of social pain, and vice versa (Eisenberger, 2012). Finally, as discussed earlier, some interventions that reduce physical pain, like Tylenol, can also reduce social pain (DeWall et al., 2010).

The pain of social rejection, it seems, is more than metaphorical. There are common neural regions that underpin social and physical pain, and the pain of a broken relationship may be as distressing as a physical wound. Eisenberger (2012) concludes:

These findings encourage us to think more carefully about the consequences of social rejection. For example, whereas physically hurting another individual is uniformly frowned on and typically punishable by law, rejecting someone else or inflicting social pain on someone is typically not held to the same standard. The work reviewed here suggests that our intuitions about and rules regarding social pain might be misguided and that these experiences might be just as damaging as experiences of physical pain. In fact, with regard to both mental and physical health, social pain-related experiences may be quite detrimental. For example, those who have experienced the loss of a loved one (versus those who have not) are twice as likely to develop depression, and those who have experienced social rejection are approximately 22 times more likely to develop depression and do so more quickly. Moreover, patients with somatoform pain or fibromyalgia, who experience pain with no medical explanation, report early experiences of social pain (emotional abuse, family conflict, and early parental loss), highlighting a potential link between these negative social experiences early on and later enhanced sensitivity to physical pain. Finally, although experiences of social pain are clearly distressing and hurtful in the moment, it is important to remember that these painful feelings after social exclusion or broken social relationships also serve a valuable function, namely, to ensure the maintenance of close social ties. (p. 133)

The Mu-Opioid System: The Brain's Natural Painkillers

As we have touched on above, the μ-opioid system can alleviate both physical and social pain. Opioid binding to μ-receptors has a reinforcing effect. It is part of the system responsible for addictions like that to morphine, but is also hypothesized to form part of the reward system that facilitates infant attachment. Studies continue to shed light on the role of μ-opioids in regulating social distress.

In 2013, a research team at the University of Michigan Molecular and Behavioral Neuroscience Institute developed an innovative methodology to test the brain's response to social pain by combining advanced brain scanning techniques (positron emission tomography, or PET) with an online dating model that incorporated scenarios of acceptance and rejection by strangers. In the study (Hsu et al., 2013) participants were asked to select people they might be interested in romantically from a wide range of photographs, just as in online dating—but then they were told these people were not interested in them! Brain activity at the moment of rejection was measured in the PET scanner and the results showed that the brain areas most active at this point were the same areas involved in physical pain. The personality of the participants proved a significant variable—for example, people who scored highly for the resiliency trait on a personality questionnaire tended to be capable of more opioid release during social rejection, especially in the amygdala, a region of the brain involved in emotional processing.

The importance of these findings is not merely theoretical; rather, they open up new lines of research in treating anxiety and depression, such as developing non-addictive medications. As Hsu noted in comments on the research, "Increasing evidence for the neural overlap of physical and social pain suggests a significant opportunity to bridge research in the treatment of chronic pain with the treatment of psychiatric disorders." The area remains rich with possibilities.

"I'm here to interview. How gentle is the corporate culture?"

FIBROMYALGIA

Fibromyalgia is a condition characterized by chronic and widespread pain and pain response to pressure (Hawkins, 2013; Ngian, Guymer, & Littlejohn, 2011) as well as fatigue, cognitive dysfunctions such as poor concentration and memory (Clauw, 2014; Glass, 2006; Hawkins, 2013), paraesthesia (Hawkins, 2013), bowel disturbances (Wallace & Hallegua, 2002), muscle spasms, and sleep disturbances (Cherney & Holland, 2016). Other symptoms can include depression and anxiety. It is estimated that fibromyalgia may affect 2–8% of the population (Chakrabarty & Zoorob, 2007, Clauw, 2014)—many cases go undiagnosed (Clauw, Arnold & McCarberg, 2011), while a far greater number of females are affected than males (Hawkins, 2013).

The legitimacy of the condition has historically been the subject of controversy among medical professionals, because the core symptoms are largely subjective and therefore not readily measured. However, the stigma is slowly disappearing as the profession accepts that it simply doesn't yet have the objective means to test some complex conditions. In the early 1800s it was classified as a rheumatoid disorder, until the discovery of tender points in the 1820s led doctors to believe that the pain was a result of systemic inflammation. In 1976, the condition was renamed fibromyalgia—a blending of the Latin "fibro" (fibrous tissue) with the Greek "myo" (muscle) and "algos" (pain) (Higuera, 2016).

The cause of fibromyalgia remains largely a mystery, although it is now believed to be a disorder not of the musculoskeletal system but of the perception of pain by the central nervous system. The idea of "central sensitization" (Hawkins, 2013) postulates that sufferers of fibromyalgia have a lower than normal threshold of pain due to nerves with a higher sensitivity to pain in the central nervous system (Ngian et al., 2011). Physical or psychological stressors can trigger abnormalities in stress and inflammatory pathways, resulting in a hypersensitivity that modulates mood (Maletic & Raison, 2009) and amplifies pain due to hyper-excitable pain processing and underactive pain-inhibiting pathways.

Although there is no single, simple approach to managing fibromyalgia (Okifuji & Hare, 2013), lifestyle plays an important part in treatment. Exercise and healthy sleep habits in particular can reduce pain and tiredness (Busch, Barber, Overend, Peloso, & Schachter, 2007; Gowans & deHueck 2004). Hydrotherapy, yoga, or tai chi can be a gentle introduction to exercise. Meditation, massage therapy, psychotherapy, biofeedback, and acupuncture have also proven helpful for some individuals. The right diet is critical to limit inflammation in the body, and a healthy whole-food diet is often recommended. Seeing an experienced naturopath can highlight areas of an individual's biochemistry that need attention and dietary changes that need to be made. Over-the-counter pain relievers can also be helpful, as can antidepressants (Häuser, Bernardy, Uçeyler & Sommer, 2009). As usual, it is advisable to seek the advice of a medical doctor when using pharmaceuticals.

DEPRESSION

> How weary, stale, flat, and unprofitable
> Seem to me all the uses of this world!
>
> *Hamlet* – William Shakespeare

What Is Depression?

Depression comes under the umbrella of mood or affective disorders, in which individuals have difficulty controlling mood states. *The Diagnostic and Statistical Manual of Mental Disorders* (5th ed.; *DSM–5*; American Psychiatric Association, 2013) categorizes depressive disorders principally as follows:

- Disruptive Mood Dysregulation Disorder
- Major Depressive Disorder
- Persistent Depressive Disorder (Dysthymia)
- Premenstrual Dysphoric Disorder
- Substance/Medication-Induced Depressive Disorder

The manual also considers depressive states arising from medical conditions such as stroke, traumatic brain injury, Parkinson's disease, and others, with two further categories covering other specified and unspecified depressive disorders (American Psychiatric Association, 2013). To keep it simple, we will limit our focus here mainly to major depressive disorder (MDD).

Depression is marked by a deep sense of sadness and reduced motivation and activity levels. Most people suffering a bout of major depression experience a recovery phase—within 3 months for 40% of sufferers, and within a year for 80%. But some suffer chronic depression (dysthymia) that persists for years (American Psychiatric Association, 2013). Factors that influence risk and prognosis are temperament, environmental factors such as adverse childhood experiences and stressful life events, genetics, and physiological factors. According to the World Health Organization, depression affects an estimated 350 million people globally (WHO, 2016).

Major Depressive Disorder Diagnostic Criteria (abbreviated from the *DSM–5*)

A. Five (or more) of the following symptoms have been present during the same 2-week period and represent a change from previous functioning; at least one of the symptoms is either (1) depressed mood or (2) loss of interest or pleasure.

1. Depressed mood most of the day, nearly every day, as indicated by either subjective report or observation made by others.
2. Markedly diminished interest or pleasure in all, or almost all, activities most of the day, nearly every day.
3. Significant weight loss when not dieting or weight gain (e.g., a change of more than 5% of body weight in a month), or decrease or increase in appetite nearly every day.
4. Insomnia or hypersomnia nearly every day.
5. Psychomotor agitation or retardation nearly every day (observable by others).
6. Fatigue or loss of energy nearly every day.
7. Feelings of worthlessness or excessive or inappropriate guilt (which may be delusional) nearly every day.
8. Diminished ability to think or concentrate, or indecisiveness, nearly every day.
9. Recurrent thoughts of death (not just fear of dying), recurrent suicidal ideation without a specific plan, or a suicide attempt or a specific plan for committing suicide.

B. The symptoms cause clinically significant distress or impairment in social, occupational, or other important areas of functioning.

C. The episode is not attributed to the physiological effects of a substance or to another medical condition.

D. The occurrence of the major depressive episode is not better explained by schizoaffective disorder, schizophrenia, schizophreniform disorder, delusional disorder, or other specified and unspecified schizophrenia spectrum and other psychotic disorders.

E. There has never been a manic episode or a hypomanic episode.

(American Psychiatric Association, 2013)

Brain Regions Involved in Depression

There are a number of brain regions implicated in affect regulation that can play a role in depressive disorders. They include the prefrontal cortex, anterior cingulate cortex, hippocampus, amygdala, and nucleus accumbens (Davidson, 2000, Davidson, Pizzagalli, Nitschke, & Putnam 2002; Grawe, 2007; Kandel, Schwartz, Jessell, Siegelbaum, & Hudspeth, 2012; Lambert & Kinsley, 2004). We will look at these areas, as well as the role of the lateral habenula and brain stem, in depression.

The Prefrontal Cortex in Depression

The prefrontal cortex (PFC) plays a dominant role in the determination of personality and temperament, guiding our behaviour on the basis of our goals and values. The PFC hemispheres appear to have different functions in this respect, with the left PFC tending towards positive goals and emotions in the form of an "approach" orientation while the right PFC specializes in avoidance goals and negative emotions (Davidson & Henriques, 2000; Grawe, 2007). Individuals with greater activation of the left PFC can experience more positive emotions in general than those whose right PFC predominates.

Depression often entails a generally underactive PFC, with hypoactivity more pronounced on the left than the right (Davidson et al., 2002). This results in a deficit of positive feelings and approach-orientated goal seeking accompanied by a surplus of negative ruminations. Processing of reward and punishment is also lateralized across the hemispheres of the PFC, with the left responding more strongly to rewards and the right to punishment. A study by Henriques and Davidson (2000) demonstrated that depressed individuals doing tasks that yielded rewarding, neutral, or punishing outcomes did not respond to rewards, whereas the control subjects did. This propensity to respond to punishment but not reward poses serious problems when trying to establish positive goals and rewards for depressed clients. However, this may be overcome by raising the overall level of activation of the PFC, thereby increasing reward processing. Antidepressant therapy has been found to increase dorsolateral PFC activity (Fales et al., 2009) and may be the most expedient way to get clients to engage in rewarding approach goals. This may not be the case, however, if there is a significant and habitual dominance of the right PFC over the left—pharmacological treatment with serotonin reuptake inhibitors (SSRI) has shown poor outcomes (Grawe, 2007).

The hypoactivation of the PFC that is typical in depression is also associated with reduced grey-matter volume along with volume decreases in the anterior cingulate cortex, orbital frontal cortex (Bora, Fornito, Panetlis, & Yücel, 2011; Grieve, Korgaonkar, Koslow,

Gordon, & Williams, 2013), and glia cells (Grawe, 2007). These findings raise the question of cause and effect: Does reduced volume in these areas cause depression, or is it a result of being depressed? Is the decreased PFC blood flow and metabolism causing the reduced volume, or is it the other way around? As yet we don't know.

A recent study on childhood depression found that depression in this stage was associated with markedly increased rates of cortical volume loss and thinning across the entire cortex in comparison with the brains of non-depressed children (Luby et al., 2016). The study found that synaptic pruning of grey matter was particularly vigorous in adolescents who had experienced symptoms of depression during their childhood. In fact the researchers found marked decreases in the right hemisphere with only marginal effects in the left—a seeming paradox given that right dominance has been associated with depression. Whatever the case, it is certain that individuals who have undergone substantial change of this kind in the neural architecture will struggle to match the capacity of healthy individuals to motivate themselves toward approach-oriented behaviour.

The Anterior Cingulate Cortex in Depression

The anterior cingulate cortex (ACC) is an important area relaying information from the limbic regions to the PFC, providing integration for visceral, attentional, and affective information for self-regulation and adaptability (Thayer & Lane, 2000). The ACC is involved in attentional processing, and especially so when there is a high demand for the attention of executive functions as the individual is faced with conflicting demands, motivations, and uncertainty (Grawe, 2007). When confronted with such difficult situations, the ACC ensures the right processing resources are made available: if things are not going the way we would like them to—producing a neural state of inconsistency—the ACC recruits areas

Some Brain Areas Involved in Depression

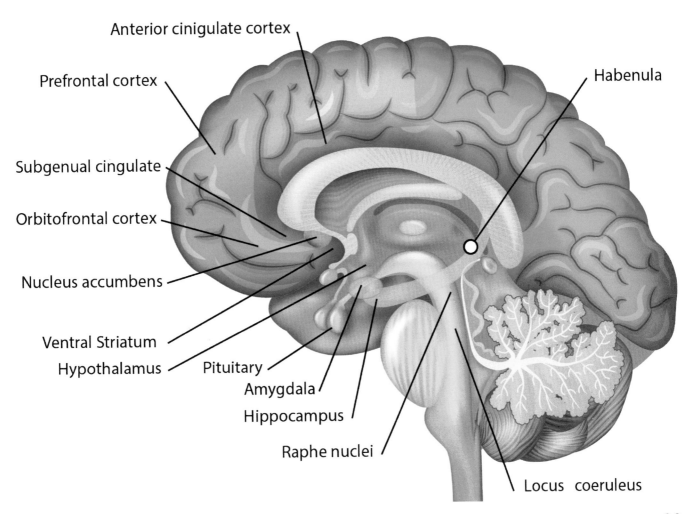

Anterior cingulate cortex
Prefrontal cortex
Habenula
Subgenual cingulate
Orbitofrontal cortex
Nucleus accumbens
Ventral Striatum
Hypothalamus   Pituitary
Amygdala
Hippocampus
Raphe nuclei
Locus coeruleus

such as the PFC to resolve such inconsistencies (Grawe, 2007).

In simplistic terms, depressed individuals have a chronically underactivated ACC, so that insufficient effort is made to recruit other brain resources when things are going wrong and something needs to be done about it. The demands of the environment can quickly overwhelm the individual whose ACC is not calling into action the right neural resources.

The ACC can be divided into two different functional areas: (a) the affect subdivision, encompassing the rostral and ventral areas connected with limbic and paralimbic regions—involved in regulating responses to stressful events, emotional expression, and social behaviour; and (b) the cognitive subdivision, comprising the dorsal regions closely connected with the dorsolateral prefrontal cortex—involved in processing cognitively demanding information (Davidson et al., 2002). Hypoactivation of the affect subdivision may blunt emotional experiencing and arousal, while hypoactivation of the cognitive subdivision may impair the recruitment and monitoring of executive functions to meet challenges.

Davidson et al. (2002) hypothesized that there may be two broad subtypes of depression, an ACC-subtype and a PFC-subtype:

The ACC-subtype may be reflected phenomenologically in a deficit in the "will-to-change", as such patients would not experience the conflict between their current state and the demands of everyday life. The PFC-subtype may fully experience such conflict and experience pronounced distress because the experience of the conflict between one's current state and the demands of everyday life are not sufficient to activate PFC-based mechanisms to organize and guide behaviour toward the resolution of the conflict. (p. 555)

The Amygdala in Depression

The amygdala is continually evaluating all incoming information for its importance to our safety and motivational goals and directing our attention toward those things with the highest emotional–motivational salience (Grawe, 2007). Because uncertainly can spell danger, the amygdala is particularly alert to uncertain and surprising information. A meta-analysis of studies on amygdala volume in MDD (Hamilton, Siemer, & Gotlib, 2008) found that medicated depressed individuals had significantly increased amygdala volume relative to healthy persons, whereas unmedicated depressed individuals showed a decrease in amygdala volume. The authors hypothesized that antidepressant-mediated increases in levels of brain-derived neurotrophic factor promoted neurogenesis—protecting the amygdala against glucocorticoid toxicity—but not in unmedicated

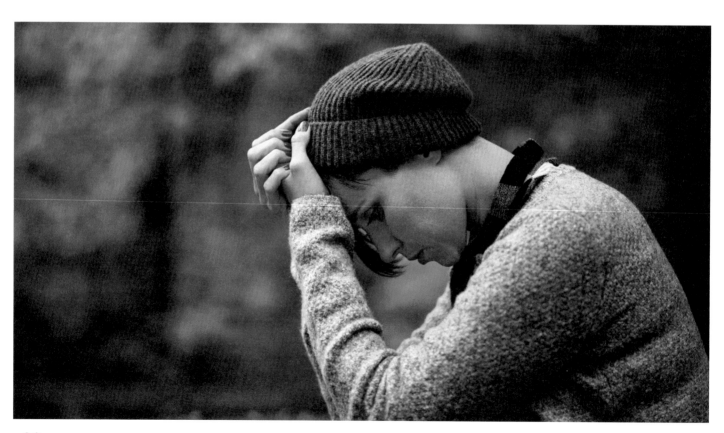

cases of depression. In a more recent review (Schmaal et al., 2016), out of 1,728 MDD patients there was found to be a trend toward smaller amygdala overall.

The Hippocampus in Depression

The hippocampus has been found to have reduced volume in individuals with MDD, with the scale of reduction apparently corresponding to the duration of depressive states (Davidson et al., 2002; Grawe, 2007). Reduction in hippocampal volume is also a feature of bipolar disorder, anxiety disorders, obsessive–compulsive disorder, PTSD, and schizophrenia (Bremner et al., 1997; Buehlmann et al., 2010; Fusar-Poli et al., 2007; Geuze, Vermetten, & Bremner, 2005; Kempton et al., 2011; Shepherd, Laurens, Matheson, Carr, & Green, 2012). It may be that such reductions in hippocampal volume are a result of enduring stress. The hippocampus contains many glucocorticoid receptors and is therefore sensitive to stress hormones like cortisol. Chronically elevated cortisol levels due to sustained stress may result in the loss of neurons and glia in all the conditions noted above. However, it is possible that a reduced hippocampus exists prior to, and facilitates, depressive and anxiety disorders. More longitudinal studies are needed to establish a clearer cause-and-effect model.

The hippocampus is also involved in the hypothalamic–pituitary–adrenal (HPA) axis stress response. It normally provides negative feedback to the HPA axis to slow the release of cortisol in the stress response, but this capacity can be overridden and is compromised in the case of sustained stress and chronically elevated levels of cortisol damage, so that a harmful continuation of cortisol release continues.

The hippocampus is important for putting things in context and helping us to respond to events by regulating our emotions accordingly (Grawe, 2007). It plays a critical part in establishing a link between the memory of contextual information and whatever we are currently faced with. For example, the war veteran who hears a car backfiring engages his hippocampus to put the sound in context (hometown as opposed to Afghanistan), which helps him to make a situation-appropriate response (keep walking down the street as opposed to hitting the deck and calling for backup). In depressed individuals the hippocampus may not be helping to regulate emotional responses in a context-appropriate way, resulting in overly exaggerated or diminished responses.

A recent meta-analysis of brain alterations in MDD concluded that the hippocampus plays a key role in the pathophysiology of MDD and that hippocampal volume reduction is evident in both recurrent and early-onset MDD (Schmaal et al., 2016).

The Nucleus Accumbens in Depression

The nucleus accumbens (NAc), like the hippocampus, helps us respond to a changing environment in an appropriate and adaptive manner. It acts as a relay between the limbic and basal ganglia structures and is involved in motivation and behavioural responses—reinforcing hunger and pleasurable activities such as sex. Given that depression is marked by a diminished interest or pleasure in things that should be pleasurable (known as *anhedonia*), it is reasonable to assume that the NAc may play a role in depression (Naranjo, Tremblay, & Busto, 2001).

A recent study on adolescent depression and early-life stress found that NAc hyporeactivity was associated with a depressed adolescence (Goff et al., 2013). For someone who is unable to experience rewards, there is little motivation to change behaviour toward rewarding goals. The NAc acts as an important integrative hub for reward-mediated behaviours and may be adversely affected by chronic stress (Heshmati & Russo, 2015). An experiment applying deep-brain stimulation to the nucleus accumbens demonstrated an anti-anxiety effect in depressed patients (Bewernick et al., 2010).

The Habenula in Depression

The habenula is involved in multiple tasks such as reproductive behaviour, stress responses, pain processing, reward processing (especially in regard to negative rewards; Matsumoto & Hikosaka, 2007), and prediction errors (Bromberg-Martin & Hikosaka, 2011). It is extensively connected to the dorsal and medial raphe nuclei—a serotonergic region—and to the ventral tegmental area—a dopaminergic region. Studies of the lateral habenula that show heightened activity when rewards are withheld have led to the idea of a "disappointment circuit".

Increased activity and reduced volume in the lateral habenula seem to be implicated with MDD, which may have functional consequences for the depressed person's ability to deal effectively with negative events (Savitz et al., 2011). Non-human studies have found that high lateral habenula activity promotes behavioural avoidance via the down-regulation of the serotonergic, noradrenergic, and dopaminergic systems and stimulation of the HPA axis. Habenula hyperactivity may influence the way we process motivationally important stimuli and result in abnormal emotional experiences and behaviours (Lawson et al., 2017; Stamatakis & Stuber, 2012)

The Brainstem in Depression

The dorsal raphe nucleus, as mentioned above, houses serotonergic (5-HT) neural networks that project into a host of brain regions including the PFC. This part of the brainstem has a huge impact on the central nervous system, as it projects serotonin pathways across the brain, releasing serotonin to mediate many processes including body temperature, blood pressure, respiration, hormone release, attention and arousal, uterine activities, aggression, food intake, sleep, and dreaming (Lambert & Kinsley, 2004).

For a long time it has been suspected that serotonin plays a role in depression and suicide. In a post-mortem study of mood disorders and suicide, it was found that those who had been diagnosed with MDD generally had a reduced dorsal raphe nucleus, yet suicide was associated with an increased dorsal raphe nucleus with a higher density but decreased size of serotonergic neurons (Matthews & Harrison, 2012). There is evidence that this seat of serotonergic activity is important in depression, but such post-mortem studies are rife with confounding variables, with only modest alterations in dorsal raphe nucleus morphology.

Another area of the brainstem that has an equally important impact on the rest of the central nervous system is the locus coeruleus (LC)—a major site for the synthesis of norepinephrine—which projects into the cortical, subcortical, and limbic structures (Malenka, Nestler, & Hyman, 2009). The LC noradrenergic system helps maintain vigilance in our responses to the environment and maintains arousal, attention, sleep–wake cycles, memory, and cognitive control, as well as playing a role in neuroplasticity and emotional responses (Benarroch, 2009). It is thought that the LC is overactive in MDD, and that antidepressants down-regulate the LC and its norepinephrine output while increasing serotonergic function (Ressler & Nemeroff, 2000). The big picture for depression, however, is complex, involving the modulation of many brain networks and neurochemicals. In the following half of this section we examine the role of neurochemicals, genetics, and neuroplasticity, to piece together a more accurate and holistic understanding of how depression affects the individual.

Neurochemicals in Depression

Evidence has mounted since the 1950s that serotonergic systems play a major role in depression. Central to this understanding early on was the observation that raising the level of serotonin appeared to reduce the symptoms of depression. The "monoamine hypothesis" of depression suggests that a deficiency in monoamines, including serotonin, causes the symptoms of depression. On the surface this logic appears reasonable, but it does not necessarily explain causality.

Early experimental evidence supported the serotonin depletion hypothesis. For example, there were found to be fewer serotonin transporter sites on platelets in depressed patients (Healy & Leonard, 1987), and less metabolic product (5-HTAA, from the breakdown of serotonin) was observed in cerebrospinal fluid (Cheetham, Katona, & Horton, 1991). But just to complicate matters, other studies have found no evidence of reduced serotonergic function in depressed patients (Gjerris, 1988). However, the monoamine hypothesis received support in the form of observations that the drug reserpine, which depletes monoamines, seemed to increase depressive symptoms. Armed with this knowledge, researchers looked at how to selectively increase synaptic serotonin levels, which led to the creation of selective serotonin reuptake inhibitors (SSRIs).

During the 1970s and 1980s, there was also a focus on monoamine receptors and how receptor density and sensitivity changed in response to different therapies, especially antidepressants. Generally the body of research supported the hypothesis that depression is marked by impaired serotonergic and adrenergic activity, with effective drug therapy increasing one or both of these systems (Palazidou, 2012). We know that presynaptic serotonergic cells have autoreceptors that monitor the amount of serotonin released by the cell. These receptors regulate the amount of serotonin release in tandem with the reuptake transporters that take serotonin from the synaptic cleft and back into the presynaptic cell. Antidepressants, by blocking reuptake mechanisms and forcing more monoamines to stay in the synaptic cleft, increase the serotonergic activity of cells in a matter of days, and autoreceptors quickly adapt to the increase in serotonin. The firing rate of the monoaminergic neurons is initially decreased to compensate for the increase in circulating monoamines, but the inhibition diminishes over time, and a therapeutic effect is felt by the patient (Lambert & Kinsley, 2005).

Another theory linking neurochemicals and depression rests on the catecholamine hypothesis introduced by Joseph Schildkraut (1965). This theory postulates that depression is a result of norepinephrine (NE) deficiency, and that an overabundance of NE leads to manic states. Although SSRIs had already produced clinically significant results in dealing with depression, the notion of a relationship between depleted NE and depression was supported by research (Delgado & Moreno, 2000; Nemeroff, 1998). It is worth noting that, as in the case of serotonin, NE depletion does not induce clinical depression in healthy people—the cause of depression appears to be more complex than simple imbalances in these levels. It is likely that depression may be a result of dysfunction in brain areas modulated by monoamine systems. The same probably holds for the involvement of another monoamine, dopamine, which has also been implicated in depression and anhedonia (Treadway & Zald, 2011).

Genetics in Depression

The early dominance of the monoamine hypothesis, which postulates that depressive symptoms are the result of decreased serotonin, noradrenalin, and possibly dopamine, has given way to alternative theories that consider neural dysfunction and genetic factors. In fact, a meta-analysis of major depression in twins concluded that the disorder is a familial one, albeit complex, arising from the combined effect of genetic and environmental influences (Sullivan, Neale, & Kendler, 2000). Epigenetic studies have been investigating how individual environmental factors modulate gene expression in depression. For instance, the 3A serotonin genotype (HTR3A-42C>T) is associated with grey-matter loss in the hippocampus and PFC in depressed individuals who have experienced early-

Serotonergic projections emanating from raphé nuclei in the brainstem and projecting across the brain

Norepinephrine projections emanating from the locus coeruleus in the brainstem.

Dopamine projections emanating from the brainstem, including the substantia nigra (SN) into the caudate nucleus.

Is the low-serotonin theory of depression wrong?

The theory that depression is strongly correlated with low levels of serotonin has dominated our approach to treatment, leading to the preeminence of SSRIs to maintain higher levels of serotonin in the synaptic cleft (rather than having the neurotransmitter reabsorbed into the postsynaptic cell). However, a new perspective has been proposed by the authors of a recent paper in *Neuroscience & Biobehavioral Reviews* (Andrews, Bharwani, Lee, Fox, & Thomson, 2015). The paper, "Is Serotonin an Upper or a Downer? The Evolution of the Serotonergic System and Its Role in Depression and the Antidepressant Response", makes three major claims about the role of serotonin in depression:

1. Serotonin is elevated in states of depression;
2. The serotonergic system is an energy regulator, and SSRIs disrupt energy homeostasis, often worsening symptoms of depression;
3. Symptom reduction is not achieved directly by the action of SSRIs but rather the brain's compensatory response to restore homeostasis.

The authors of this paper say there are problems with the low serotonin hypothesis, including the following:

- Alternative drugs that block serotonin reuptake are not effective in treating depression.
- Early studies of reserpine-induced depression may have been flawed, and reserpine may actually have antidepressant properties.
- SSRIs can increase serotonin levels in minutes to hours, but the therapeutic effect takes weeks of treatment.
- Serotonin reduction in the non-depressed individual does not replicate depressive symptoms.
- Neonatal exposure to SSRIs causes depressive symptoms in adult rodents.
- Genetic manipulation to increase synaptic serotonin is associated with increased depressive symptoms.
- Antidepressants are only modestly more effective than placebos.

The serotonergic system is involved in a vast number of functions beyond mood, possibly across every major system, organ, and metabolic process. Essentially, Andrews et al. (2015) argued that serotonin is involved in key areas of energy regulation, and that it is important to maintain a homeostatic equilibrium of serotonin levels when there are metabolically costly processes occurring When SSRIs upset the balance of extracellular serotonin, the brain has to work hard to elicit a compensatory response to restore energy homeostasis. This raises the question: Is it possible that serotonin is not the key to depression but a distal factor in the causal pathway for the condition? Serotonin is likely an important part of regulating energy-intensive states like depression, but the solution for depression may not be a simple matter of artificially tipping the balance of serotonin across the entire system.

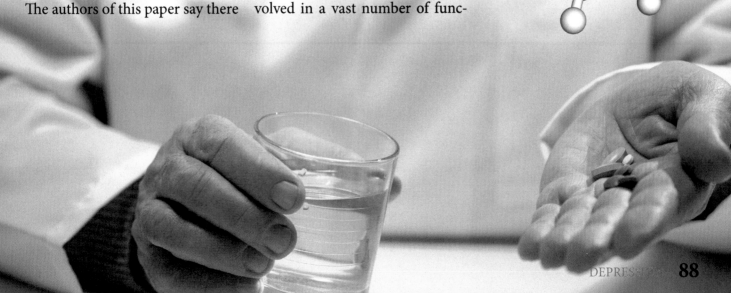

Stressed Rhesus Monkeys
and the Serotonin Transporter Gene

Studies on rhesus monkeys that investigated the impact of attachment (Suomi, 1999, as cited in Grawe, 2007) yielded some telling results: monkeys raised with peers, but without mothers, tended to be more impulsive and aggressive and drank more alcohol (made available as part of the experiment) as young adults than their peers. They also had lower levels of serotonin metabolite (5-HIAA) and higher glucose metabolism in their brains, making them hyper-aroused. These monkeys, with very poor attachment experiences, developed a biological system shaped by insecure attachment.

The researchers found that monkeys growing up without mothers had chronically lower serotonin levels, significantly affecting their social relationships and the capacity of female monkeys to be good mothers themselves. There seems to be a positive correlation between attachment relationships and serotonin levels that can have a calming effect on neural firing—animals with more serotonin available appear to do better socially.

The truly groundbreaking finding of these types of studies (see, e.g., Bennett, Abee, & Henrickson, 1998; Lesch et al., 1996) concerned experience-dependent gene expression: monkeys with poor attachment whose serotonin transporter gene (5-HTT) had the "short" HTT-allele (less efficient for expressing the gene) would have lower serotonin levels than monkeys with the "long" HTT-allele. Interestingly, monkeys with the short HTT-allele who did have normal attachment with their mothers did not have lowered serotonin levels—their genotype may have put them at genetic risk of serotonergic hypofunction, but secure attachment averted this genetic expression. On the other hand, monkeys who had the stronger genotype with the long HTT-allele, even though they may have had the disadvantage of a motherless upbringing, still had normal serotonergic functioning—their genotype protected them from the impact of not having a mother (at least in terms of serotonergic function). These findings, that favourable versus unfavourable life experiences can alter gene expression affecting areas like the serotonergic system, are important when we consider the environmental variables at play in cases of anxiety and depression.

life stress (Gatt et al., 2010). And just as we saw with the rhesus monkeys, human carriers of the 5-HTTLPR short allele are more prone to depression if they have suffered one or more earlier stressful life events, which lends further support to the idea that an individual's response to environmental stress is moderated by genetic makeup (Caspi et al., 2003; Karg, Burmeister, Shedden, & Sen, 2011).

Another line of research implicates brain-derived neurotropic factor (BDNF), which is involved in the growth of new neurons in the hippocampus and represents an important mechanism of adult brain plasticity. Stress suppresses BDNF synthesis in the hippocampus, and depressed patients have been shown to have lower serum BDNF concentrations than healthy subjects. Antidepressants and electroconvulsive therapy seem to increase BDNF serum concentrations and reduce depressive symptoms (Piccinni et al., 2009; Shimizu et al., 2003). BDNF seems a good candidate for study in depression, as BDNF genetic variations influence brain areas related to mood (Palazidou, 2012). The Met allele BDNF genotype has been associated with abnormal secretion of BDNF, abnormal hippocampal neuronal function, and impaired episodic memory (Hariri et al., 2003) as well as smaller hippocampal volume (Frodl, Möller, & Meisenzahl, 2008). However, the evidence for the involvement of BDNF in the pathophysiology of depression is inconsistent and does not support a simple causal relationship between total brain BDNF levels and mood (Groves, 2007). Rather, the role of BDNF in modulating activity-dependent plasticity within emotional processing networks may be compromised in depression. In other words, BDNF may not control mood directly, but is critical in the process that determines how a plastic change influences mood (Castrén, Võikar, & Rantamäki, 2007).

Neuroplasticity in Depression

As discussed above, studies found that antidepressant medication rapidly increased the transmission at monoaminergic synapses, yet patients did not typically feel the therapeutic effects for some weeks after starting treatment. This points to something beyond merely the synaptic change elicited by the antidepressant. The neuroplasticity theory of depression suggests that the depressed brain has reduced plasticity in key areas such as the PFC, hippocampus, and amygdala, leading to neural and glial loss and pathology (Andrade & Rao, 2010). The theory suggests that depression is a disorder of the hardwiring of the brain rather than a chemical imbalance. In this context, antidepressants can protect against some of these neuronal architectural and connectivity changes that are at the foundation of the disorder (Castrén & Hen, 2013). Research demonstrating that stress and depression disrupt adult neurogenesis in the hippocampus, and research showing antidepres-

Brain Stimulation Treatment

Andres Lozano, from the Division of Neurosurgery at the University of Toronto, led a study in which the researchers experimented with implanting electrodes into the anterior cingulate gyrus of depressed patients who had not responded well to other forms of therapy (Lozano et al., 2008). In each of 20 patients they surgically implanted a single, fine electrode deep into the anterior cingulate gyrus where it would deliver a continuous pulse of electrical stimulation. This sort of deep-brain stimulation therapy is thought to create changes in the metabolic activity of the circuits implicated in depression—in other words, to fire up the circuits that are typically underactive in depression. The results were impressive, given that these patients had not responded to traditional treatments. Within a month following surgery, 35% of the patients had positively responded, with 10% in remission. This figure rose within 6 months after surgery, with 60% showing positive responses and 35% meeting the criteria for remission of depression—and these positive outcomes, for the most part, were maintained for 12 months with minimal adverse effects.

Subsequent studies have replicated the success of deep brain stimulation in both major depression and bipolar disorder (Holtzheimer et al., 2012; Lozano et al., 2012), potentially paving the way to more effective treatment strategies for the most difficult cases of major depression while highlighting the importance of the subcallosal cingulate gyrus in depressive symptoms.

Elements Implicated in Depression

Genetic response to environment/ past experiences

Environment

Increased Stressors

Serotonin, Norepinephrine, Dopamine (decreases)

Proinflammatory Cytokines increases

BDNF (decreases)

HPA Dysregulation (increased cortisol)

Hippocampal (atrophy)

PFC Hypoactivity (more pronounced L-PFC hypoactivity) Negative ruminations, avoidance

Anterior cingulate cortex (under-activated) Does not recruit neural resources needed to meet needs.

Limbic Hyperactivity Amygdala changes Habenula atrophy

Gut microbiota (influencing neurochemistry and immune system)

Nucleus accumbens hypoactivity (less reward mediated behaviour)

sants' increased neurogenesis in the hippocampus, also support the neuroplasticity theory (Duman & Voleti, 2012; Eisch & Petrik, 2012).

Other research substantiating the plasticity theory includes the study of psychedelic ketamine, which can alleviate depressive symptoms (Vollenweider & Kometer, 2010). Psychedelics can have a rapid antidepressant effect, and researchers such as Vollenweider and Kometer suggest that psychedelics alter glutamatergic neurotransmission in prefrontal–limbic circuits, leading to more adaptive neuroplasticity (see also Duman & Aghajanian, 2012).

Inflammation

It has been well established that the immune system is involved in the pathophysiology of major depressive disorder (Villanueva, 2013). Signalling molecules of the immune system, called proinflammatory cytokines, can elicit symptoms of anxiety and depression; typically, those with major depression will have elevated levels of circulating proinflammatory cytokines (Palazidou, 2012). It is interesting that in animal studies, researchers have been able to induce depressive-like behaviour and neutralize the effects of antidepressants by administering the proinflammatory cytokine interleukin-6 (Sukoff Rizzo et al., 2012), and people treated with interferon alpha (another cytokine) can develop depressive-like symptoms (Shelton & Miller, 2010). As the immune system activates an inflammatory response, it can deplete the body of the serotonin precursor tryptophan— a molecule that is used by the body to make serotonin. Inflammation may also influence noradrenergic activity, and it stimulates the HPA axis. Chronic physical illness or stress also releases inflammatory cytokines that can reduce glucocorticoid receptor function, which in turn can increase inflammation. In fact there are multiple causes for an inflammatory response, including obesity, multiple sclerosis, cardiovascular disease, and psoriasis (Shelton & Miller, 2010). Whatever the cause of the inflammation, it seems this process plays a role in depression.

The Gut

There is growing evidence that the interplay between the brain and the gut is of significant importance to well-being. In depression, the influence of the gut microbiota over brain chemistry and resulting behaviour is a variable we must take seriously (Villanueva, 2013). Recent studies suggest that the microbiota could activate our immune system and affect our central nervous system, delivering substances such as serotonin and gamma-aminobutyric acid (Evrensel & Ceylan, 2015). Such findings have led to the development of psychobiotic-based therapeutic strategies for mood disorders, and have directed research focus to the interplay between physical ailments such as irritable bowel syndrome and depression (Dinan & Cryan, 2013). We will examine this area in more depth in the next section of the guide, on the Brain–Body connection.

Summary of the Pathophysiology of Depression

Depression is a complex phenomenon, from the social and environmental factors that prime our stress responses and express genes in different ways, to chemical balances, inefficient neural architectures, and lack of neural plasticity. There is no single, unified theory, nor a simple solution. As psychotherapists, we should be aware first and foremost of the complexity of the neurobiological, epigenetic, and environmental factors at play, in order to have a holistic appreciation of the disorder and avoid the temptation to offer narrow solutions. Given the state of knowledge to this point, it would be wise to remain open to a range of therapeutic techniques, since clients with major depressive disorder are likely to have multiple system deficits. One technique, one drug, one therapy is unlikely to give a client the level of support he or she needs to achieve genuine transformation.

BRAIN–BODY

As a society we are becoming increasingly aware of the critical interplay between the systems of the body and mental health. Dysfunctions of the mind or body have a bidirectional effect, in ways more profound than we may have appreciated in the past. Research from the biological and psychological sciences is painting a more integrative picture of the brain–body connection than ever before. Although the connections may seem obvious—intuitive—they represent a significant change in thinking from the standard modern approach to mental health from an etiological and treatment perspective. We are now gaining a more refined understanding of the way the central nervous system (CNS) and the rest of the body modulate each other, and how this insight can contribute to better treatment and prevention of mental disorders. In this section, while we touch on some of the body systems that have an effect on our mental well-being, we are really only scratching the surface of this wonderfully complex phenomenon of the brain–body connection.

The Heart

Thinkers throughout the ages have considered the heart to be the seat of the emotions and at the centre of spiritual life. William Harvey (1578–1657), an English doctor who was the first to fully describe the circulatory system that delivers blood to the body and brain, said, "Every affection of the mind that is attended either with pain or pleasure, hope or fear, is the cause of an agitation whose influence extends to the heart" (Rosch, 2015, p. 7).

In broad terms, our contemporary view of the heart is one of a complex and interdependent relationship between the heart and mind. Early studies of heart–brain communication were intent on explaining the influence of the brain over the heart, yet we now know there is more neural "traffic" from the heart to the brain than the other way around (McCraty, 2015a). In fact the heart communicates with the brain not only through the nervous system, but also through hormones, pulse waves created by heart contractions, and the electromagnetic field generated by the heart. At the forefront of the new science of the heart–brain connection has been recent research into heart rate variability (HRV), a measure of the nervous system's flexibility for emotional self-regulation.

In the 1960s and 70s, researchers John and Beatrice Lacey established scientific evidence that the heart communicates to the brain in a way that affects how we perceive and react to the world (Lacey & Lacey, 1974). German research by Velden and Wölk in the 1980s found that cognitive performance and cortical function are under the influence of the heart by means of afferent (heart to brain) inputs on neurons in the thalamus that affect the global synchronization of cortical activity (Velden & Wölk, 1987; Wölk & Velden, 1989). Importantly, the researchers identified the pattern and stability of these afferent inputs, which in turn have global effects on brain function. The heart, it seems, wields more control over the brain than we had supposed. Since these early discoveries there has been a proliferation of studies on HRV as a marker for physical and emotional well-being.

Simply put, HRV measures the variability in time between heartbeats. This, it turns out, is a good gauge of the interplay between the autonomous nervous system (ANS) and the heart. The parasympathetic branch of the ANS, via the vagus nerve, connects to the heart's pacemaker (the concentration of nerve cells in the sinoatrial node in the heart that initiates heart contractions) and exerts an inhibitory effect on heart rate. It is, as it were, the braking system for the heart. On release of the parasympathetic brake, the heart rate rises. This operation of the vagus nerve upon the heart's pacemaker occurs on a moment-by-moment basis, resulting in slight variations of timing

The heart influences the brain through four lines of communication:

1. The nervous system
2. Hormones
3. Pulse waves
4. Electromagnetic fields

---

between heartbeats. High HRV indicates that the heart is readily and flexibly influenced by the vagal brake, and this, it has been discovered, is a good indicator of our emotional flexibility.

The Intuitive Heart

Intuition is normally conceived as a cognitive–affective understanding, or "affectively charged judgments that arise through rapid, nonconscious, and holistic associations" (Dane & Pratt, 2007, p. 33). However, there may be other types of intuitive process where the heart informs the mind in unique ways. One such possibility lies in the capacity of our nervous system to sense electromagnetic fields, which the heart both produces and is sensitive to. This is referred to as cardioelectromagnetic communication:

> The heart is the most powerful source of electromagnetic energy in the human body, producing the largest rhythmic electromagnetic field of any of the body's organs. The heart's electrical field is about 60 times greater in amplitude than the electrical activity generated by the brain. This field, measured in the form of an electrocardiogram (ECG), can be detected anywhere on the surface of the body. Furthermore, the magnetic field produced by the heart is more than 100 times greater in strength than the field generated by the brain and can be detected up to 3 feet away from the body, in all directions, using SQUID-based magnetometers. (McCraty, 2015b, p. 36)

Psychophysiologist Rollin McCraty makes a fascinating exploration of the science of the electromagnetic sensitivities of the heart, including its apparently "nonlocal" or pre-stimulus knowledge and how this is communicated to the brain, in Chapter 7 of his book *Science of the Heart: Exploring the Role of the Heart in Human Performance* (Volume 2; McCraty, 2015b). Some of the intuitive capacity of the heart may be explained in the future by quantum neurophysics (Tarlacı & Pregnolato, 2016), and much remains speculative. Nevertheless, the interplay between the heart and mind is itself intuitive to most psychotherapists—as it is to anyone who has given the advice, "Listen to your heart."

The Polyvagal Theory

The polyvagal theory was put forward by Stephen Porges (2011). It proposes three vagal-mediated adaptive responses for different circumstances, namely safety, danger, and extreme threat to life. These responses are initiated by our *perception* of what is going on in our environment.

The first of these circuits is the ventral vagal complex (also known as the "smart vagus"), which downregulates the sympathetic "fight or flight" response so we can be social, engage in bonding, and emotionally self-regulate. This part of our nervous system is implicated in social communication on account of its effect on the muscles of the face, and in self-soothing/calming through inhibition of the defensive limbic system. The ventral vagal complex also influences heart rate: high vagal tone (strength of vagus response) has a suppressant effect on the heart's natural pacemaker; in the absence of vagal regulation, the heart's pacemaker rapidly increases heart rate.

The second circuit is the dorsal vagal complex, an unmyelinated circuit that is found in most vertebrates and is associated with primitive survival strategies. This is the branch of the vagus nerve that engages defensive "fight or flight" behaviour in the face of threats.

The third vagal mechanism acts through the dorsal vagal complex, which, in the face of an extreme threat to life, will feign death by producing neurogenic bradycardia (slowing of the heart rate) via the parasympathetic nervous system, manifesting in a freeze or faint. The bradycardia can be paralleled by apnoea—a response that may be adaptive for reptiles, but is potentially lethal for humans.

As mentioned previously, the initiation of any one of these three vagal responses is based on our perception of threat. This perception Porges calls *neuroception*—a subconscious neural process that distinguishes whether situations or people are safe, dangerous, or life-threatening. If there is no perception of threat, then the ventral vagal complex has control and we can be social and relaxed; we have good HRV, and all is well. But we all have different perceptions, or subconscious neuroceptions, about what is threatening and what is not, based on earlier experiences. For an individual who has had mainly experiences of trauma, nothing in the world feels safe, and the default response is characterized by more frequent engagement of the dorsal vagal complex than is necessary to ensure actual safety. Lower HRV has been observed in individuals with post-traumatic stress disorder and borderline personality disorder (Meyer et al., 2016), rendering these people in a psychological state more prone to "fight or flight" than social engagement behaviours (Austin, Riniolo, & Porges, 2007).

The Gut–Brain Axis

The broad term *gut–brain axis* describes the bidirectional communication pathways of the central nervous system, the hypothalamic–pituitary–adrenal (HPA) axis, the autonomic nervous system, and the gut microbiota. Our bodies are host to an enormous population of microorganisms, collectively called microbiota or microflora, with the genomes in the microbiota termed the microbiome. These gut microbes outnumber the cells in our bodies by a factor of 10, contain 150 times more genes than our own (Gill et al., 2006; Qin et al., 2010), and comprise more than 1,000 species (Qin et al., 2010) and over 7,000 strains (Ley, Peterson, & Gordon, 2006). A growing body of research implicates the gut microbiome in the regulation of the CNS and behaviour in general. What we might term the microbiome-gut–brain axis, then, is a bidirectional communication network between the brain and gut modulated by neurochemicals and microbiota (Mawe & Hoffman, 2013; Mayer, 2011; Rhee, Pothoulakis, & Mayer, 2009).

Important findings in this research include that the microbial content of the gut is critical to the normal development of the HPA axis, brain-derived neurotrophic factor (BDNF, a key neurotrophin involved in neuronal growth), and expression of NMDA receptors in the cortex and hippocampus (Sudo et al., 2004). A number of studies have investigated changes in gene expression in the brains of "germ-free" mice—mice raised in a way that has significantly reduced their gut microbiota—finding decreased hippocampal expression of BDNF, which is important for brain plasticity, and alterations in normal neurotransmitter signalling (Mayer, Knight, Mazmanian, Cryan, & Tillisch, 2014).

The vagal complex modulates bodily emotional responses.

There are several ways the gut microbiome influences the CNS, through humoral and neural routes (Bravo et al., 2011; Cryan & O'Mahony, 2011), and through neurotransmitter modulation such as elevating plasma tryptophan—a precursor to serotonin (Desbonnet, Garrett, Clarke, Bienenstock, & Dinan, 2008). But the influence is not unidirectional. The CNS can change gastrointestinal motility, secretion, and intestinal permeability—actions that alter the gut environment for resident bacteria (Rhee et al., 2009). Stress can also induce permeability of the gut, allowing bacteria to cross the epithelial barrier, initiating a mucosal immune response that changes the composition of the microbiome (Kiliaan et al., 1998).

Researchers have been examining how to support the gut microbiome for normal brain function and experimenting with treatment for CNS disorders, in particular by the introduction of probiotics (Grenham, Clarke, Cryan, & Dinan, 2011). But this is a complex field involving not only many different species and strains of bacteria that elicit different effects in the gut, but neurochemicals and the CNS. It is a complexity we are only just starting to unravel. Nevertheless, the health of the gut plays a critical role in mental well-being, and psychotherapists would be well advised to make referrals to naturopaths or other professionals who can treat possible imbalances in the gut when necessary.

The Immune System

As we saw in the previous section on depression, the immune system is implicated in psychopathology, with inflammation being an important variable in major depression (Haapakoski, Mathieu, Ebmeier, Alenius, & Kivimäki, 2015). There is bidirectional communication between the brain and the immune system via many specialized pathways, such as the release of inflammatory cytokines in response to illness or other stressors. Cytokines can alter the function of serotonin, dopamine, and glutamate in the brain, which play critical roles in depression. Stressful life experiences such as complex trauma may trigger long-lasting and systemic inflammatory responses. Childhood trauma can trigger such a response, affecting brain development and ultimately posing a risk of psychopathology (Danese & Baldwin, 2017).

Animal studies have found that psychological stress is communicated from the CNS to the immune system and from the immune system to back to the brain, releasing immune cells from the bone marrow. These immune cells, called monocytes, are released into circulation and provide inflammatory signals to the brain, with the potential to induce anxiety-like behaviour (McKim et al., 2016). These findings suggest that inflammation-reducing therapies could be an effective strategy for patients with anxiety and depression. Inflammation is a response that can be initiated by a multitude of variables including pathogens, stress, diet, and chemicals, all of which can prompt the release of inflammatory cy-

Healthy CNS function   Alterations in behaviour, cognition, emotions

Normal Gut   Abnormal Gut

Physiological levels of inflammatory cells/mediators. Normal gut microbiota.

Increased levels of inflammatory cells/mediators. Intestinal dysbiosis.

Brain–gut–microbe in health and disease (adapted from Grenham, Clarke, Cryan, & Dinan, 2011). A stable gut microbiota helps establish normal gut physiology and appropriate signalling from the gut to the central nervous system. Poor gut microbiota health leads to inappropriate brain–gut axis signalling and negative CNS states. Stress signals originating from the CNS also negatively impact gut function and microbiota.

tokines. The consumption of some foods, such as refined sugars, caffeine, alcohol, and anything triggering an allergic response, can initiate inflammation. There are also environmental and lifestyle factors, such as exposure to toxic metals, pesticides, herbicides, chronic stress, nutritional deficiencies, poor sleep, and ongoing infections, to name just a few. The cytokines released in an inflammatory response can cause oxidative stress to cells and shunt the serotonin precursor tryptophan toward the production of quinolinate, an excitotoxin in the CNS, which can lead to hindered neuronal function or apoptotic death (Guillemin, 2012).

There is still much to learn about the interplay of inflammation and mental health, but it is safe to assume that any chronic inflammation equates to a state of stress that is detrimental both developmentally and for our ultimate well-being.

The Following Strategies Can Help Reduce Inflammation*

- Exercise—20 to 30 minutes of exercise at a minimum of 3 times per week.
- Rest—practise good sleep hygiene and get enough sleep.
- Stress Management—use relaxation techniques you enjoy; include deep-breathing exercises.
- Diet—focus on omega-3 fatty acids, alkaline-producing content, and whole foods rather than refined foods. Avoid saturated fats.

*Consult relevant professionals for exercise and diet strategies.

MEMORY

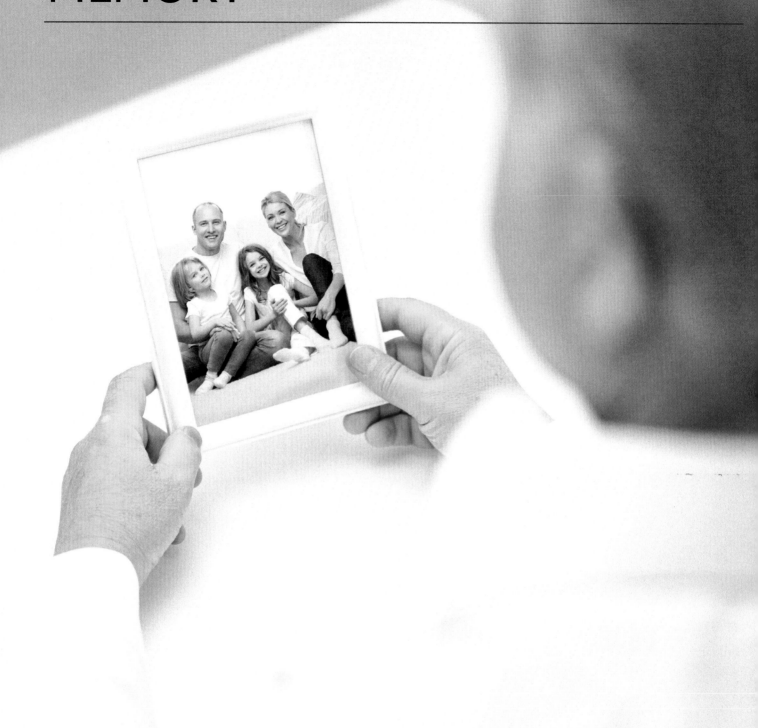

All through our lives we are on an insatiable learning quest that we call memory. We continually store information, either consciously or unconsciously, and draw on that learning to be animated and have a sense of who we are and what the world is. It is a never-ending cycle of encoding, storage, and retrieval (Baddeley, Eysenck, & Anderson, 2009). When you think about it, this process of encoding and storing experience as memory is everything to us. We are born into the world ready to learn, ready to memorize, and in fact have already started the learning quest in the womb (Partanen et al., 2013). Without memory you cannot talk, walk, or move in any meaningful way; you would know no past; you would have no concept of self or place—no concept of who you are, where you are, or what surrounds you. From the unconscious reflexes and motor control that allow you to walk with little conscious effort to the complexities of advanced cognition such as solving equations in theoretical physics, memory is the indispensable operant. Memory links our past with our present and allows us to project into the future—it absolutely influences our next move. Our lives, and the memories our lives are built on, are uniquely crafted by the complex interplay of our individual neural architecture and genetic expression immersed in the experience of our environment.

The epigenetic process—where our experience of the environment alters the way in which genes are expressed— is another fascinating aspect of memory. But it is a complex subject, and too large for our brief study of memory here (for a study on epigenetics for therapists, see Peckham, 2013). For now, our focus here are the networks and molecules involved in memory encoding, storage, and retrieval.

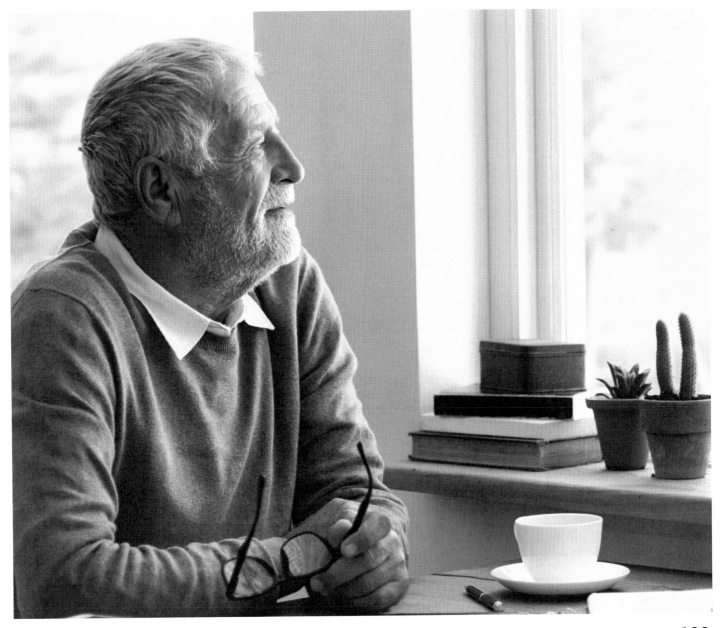

Ever since Paul Broca, in 1861, discovered that damage to a particular part of the left frontal lobe (now known as Broca's area) produced deficits in language, there has been a quest to discover the discrete parts of the brain that mediate specific cognitive functions, including in this quest the prevailing question: "Are there discrete brain systems devoted to memory?" Certainly, in the last few decades, there has been significant progress in our understanding of learning and memory. Eric Kandel, who received the Nobel Prize for his research on memory, and whose outstanding career and discoveries are documented in his book *In Search of Memory: The Emergence of a New Science of Mind* (Kandel, 2006), is perhaps the foremost of the many researchers who have given us a much more sophisticated understanding of memory processes. Kandel's work, famously with the elegant sea slug *Aplysia californica*, has uncovered some of the secrets of learning and memory, most notably the mechanisms of memory consolidation and neural plasticity. Kandel identified two problems: the *systems* problem of memory (Where in the brain is memory stored?) and the *molecular* problem of memory (What are the mechanisms of this storage?).

When addressing the systems problem we can divide memory into two broad categories:

1. **Short-term memory**—momentary memory that is processed in the temporal lobe and hippocampus before being transferred into long-term memory or discarded. This transient memory can also be manipulated by the prefrontal cortex—a process known as *working memory* (a distinction can be made between short-term and working memory, see Aben, Stapert, & Blokland, 2012)—before it is either lost or integrated into long-term memory. Short-term memory can be thought of as a transient representation of goal-relevant knowledge (Kandel, Schwartz, Jessell, Siegelbaum, & Hudspeth, 2012), an important part of our consciousness. We can further divide short-term memory into verbal and visuospatial information that is coordinated by *executive control processes* that allocate attention to the different memory systems.

2. **Long-term memory**—memory that can persist for years and is encoded in the cerebral cortex. Long-term memory is further divided into:

Riding a bike without having to "think about it" utilizes your procedural memory function.

a. ***Explicit (declarative) memory***—the memory of facts and events, and people, objects, and places, processed in the medial temporal lobe and hippocampus. This sort of memory requires conscious effort to recall. For example, the legendary spatial memory held in the hippocampus of London taxi drivers actually enlarges their hippocampus, full of London street information, ready for conscious recall. Explicit memory is mediated by the processes of encoding, storage, consolidation, and retrieval, and the elements of this form of memory are distributed among many brain regions that can be accessed independently (Kandel et al., 2012).

b. ***Implicit (procedural) memory***—the memory of skills and habits of the neocortex, striatum, amygdala, cerebellum, and reflex pathways that do not require conscious attention to recall. These are the memories that encode the automatic part of our behaviour—walking and talking, and all the special skills we have learnt. Implicit memory can be further categorized as:

- Priming—the improved perception of a word or object by prior experience, processed in the neocortex;

- Procedural—skills and habits processed in the striatum;

Types of Memory

Memory Type	Description	Key Brain Areas
Sensory	Neural traces from sensory input lasting less than a second	All sensory input going to specific sensory areas of the brain.
Short-term	The holding of a limited amount of information for less than about 18 seconds without manipulation or rehearsal (Revlin, 2012), and may be limited to 5–9 discrete bits of information at any one time (first proposed by Miller, 1956).	Hippocampus; subiculum
Working	A prefrontal cognitive capacity responsible for the transient holding, processing, and manipulation of information (Diamond, 2013)	Dorsolateral prefrontal cortex
Long-term explicit	The conscious memory of facts and events, also known as declarative memory; can also be divided into episodic (autobiographical events and experiences) and semantic (facts, concepts) memory.	Medial temporal lobe: perirhinal, entorhinal, and parahippocampal cortices; hippocampus
Long-term implicit	The unconscious memory of skills and tasks, also known as procedural memory; can be further divided into priming, procedural, associative learning, and non-associative learning	Neocortex (priming); striatum (procedural); amygdala (emotional responses in associative learning); cerebellum (skeletal musculature in associative learning); reflex pathways (non-associative learning)

The division of memory types below follows the Atkinson-Shiffrin model (Atkinson & Shiffrin, 1968), also known as the multi-store or modal model of memory. The Atkinson-Shiffrin model defines discrete types of processes, as opposed to the levels-of-processing model (Craik & Lockhart, 1972), which assumes a continuum of depth of mental processing, from shallow perception to deeper semantic memory.

Glossary

cyclic adenosine 3',5'-cyclic monophosphate (cAMP): An important "second messenger" for intracellular signalling, such as transferring into cells the effects of hormones that cannot pass through the plasma membrane, for the activation of protein kinases.

CRE (cAMP recognition element): A promotor element that CREB-1 binds to in a chain of interactions to promote gene transcription.

CREB-1 (cAMP response element binding protein 1): An activator-type transcription factor that stimulates transcription upon binding to the CRE—a key element involved in turning on gene transcription. In the case of memory formation, the interaction between this activator type and the repressor type (CREB-2) initiates the emergence of long-lasting synaptic enhancement, that is, memory consolidation (Wagatsuma et al., 2006).

CREB-2 (cAMP response element binding protein 2): A similar transcription factor to CREB-1 but inhibits the transcription of downstream genes. When CREB-2 is relieved of its repressive function, and CREB-1 is activated, it produces a cascade of new gene expression for the consolidation of memory.

CBP (CREB-binding protein): A CREB protein involved in transcription.

MAPK (mitogen-activated protein kinase): A protein kinase (an enzyme that modifies other proteins by adding a phosphate group to them) that is involved in many cellular responses to stimuli and regulates a number of cellular functions including gene expression.

PKA (protein kinase): An enzyme that modifies other proteins by adding a phosphate group to them, resulting in functional changes in the target proteins.

Transcription: The first step in gene expression, where segments of DNA are copied to RNA (single chain nucleotides that convey genetic information to direct synthesis of specific proteins) to produce a primary transcript followed by various modifications to yield functional forms of RNAs.

- Associative learning—classical and operant conditioning such as fear learning in the amygdala and the learning of motor skills in the cerebellum; and
- Non-associative learning—habituation and sensitization along reflex pathways (Kandel et al., 2012).

Explicit memory processing involves four related yet distinct operations (Kandel et al., 2012):

1. *Encoding.* For incoming information to be remembered it must be "well-encoded", or what might be termed "deep" encoding (Craik & Lockhart, 1972). Encoding involves attending to the new information and associating it with prior knowledge. Motivation to remember (which may involve more focused attention) is correlated with deep encoding; sleep and dreaming may also play a part in encoding memories, as the experiences of the day are processed and associations made while you sleep.

2. *Storage.* Neural mechanisms, and the resulting neural architecture, retain the learning over time—learning that may last a lifetime. There seems to be an almost unlimited capacity for long-term storage, unlike working memory that can only hold a few bits of information for a limited time.

3. *Consolidation.* Once neural connections are established to hold the memory trace, consolidation makes the connections more stable. This involves the expression of genes, protein synthesis, and changes in the synaptic connections.

4. *Retrieval.* The recall of stored memories is a constructive process that brings together the various elements of a memory and reconstructs them into a perception of the thing remembered. Recall uses a range of strategies such as comparison, inference, supposition, and guessing, and using the new information to generate, or recreate, a memory that seems coherent and consistent with our other memories and perceptions. Because memory retrieval is a constructive process it is open to distortion and also, as we will learn below, open to reconsolidation in a form different from what was originally encoded or even from what was last reconsolidated. In other words, memories can change.

What then are the mechanisms that allow the storage of memory to occur? Kandel and others have discovered that repetition is one mechanism whereby the information being received is converted from short- to long-term memory through altered gene expression and the growth of new synaptic connections. These changes, which we call *experience-dependent neuroplasticity*, require protein synthesis to create more permanent synaptic connections between neurons. When there is repeated activation of a neuron, the second messenger system within the cell causes changes in the cell nucleus, where the genes are located, and this works in distinct ways for explicit and implicit memories. Second messengers are small intracellular molecules that are produced after the first neurotransmitter has activated the receptor. Second messengers activate intracellular signaling pathways that amplify the signal and activate or inhibit transcription factors, inducing a cellular response.

It is also important to note, especially so for the psychotherapist, that one-trial learning (a single exposure to a stimulus) can happen when there is strong emotion involved—as in a traumatic event, for example. As anyone who has been traumatized by a single transient event (such as being held up at gunpoint) can attest, that one event can form a remarkably stable and enduring memory. There may, however, be cognitive processes going on after the event that persist to consolidate the memory of such a trauma.

To take an example, let us look at long-term implicit memory formation (consolidation) that involves changes in chromatin structure (the DNA double helix packaged around proteins called histones) and gene expression. The following is a somewhat simplified version, with many details and regulatory factors omitted. (Those wishing to know all the detailed interactions are encouraged to read Chapter 66 of Kandel et al., 2012.) When there is repeated activation of a set of neurons (e.g., practicing scales on the piano), there is a prolonged rise in cAMP (see Glossary) due to repeated application of serotonin. This, in turn, activates protein kinase (PKA) that does two things: first, it translocates into the cell nucleus to turn on CREB-1 to activate gene transcription while activating mitogen-activated protein kinase (MAPK), which turns off the inhibitory gene repressor CREB-2. Then, once activated, CREB-1 influences downstream genes and stimulates the growth of new synaptic connections. These new connections consolidate a memory that is lasting.

In the case of explicit (declarative) memory, repeated stimulation of neuronal circuits again establishes a

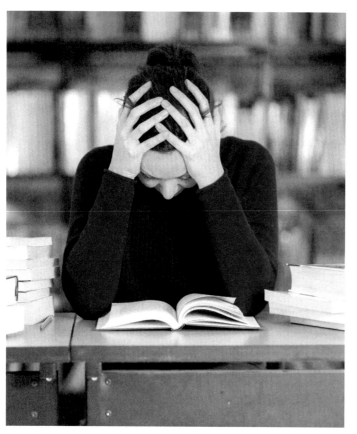

consolidated memory. Like implicit memory, explicit memory uses modulatory transmitters and CREB-mediated switches to initiate downstream gene expression to grow new synaptic connections. But unlike implicit memory, it employs NMDA receptors and the dopaminergic system to activate a cAMP/PKA pathway within the neuron, triggering the cascade of events that results in a more stable connection. (Once again, for full details on explicit memory consolidation, see Chapter 67 of Kandel et al., 2012).

Students have been known to take amphetamines or other dopamine-enhancing drugs when cramming for exams to heighten explicit consolidation by supercharging the front end of that process. The reverse is also conceivable: drugs that short-circuit the cAmp–PKA–CREB pathways may limit the consolidation of traumatic memories if administered in a timely manner. Trauma sufferers should approach the use of drugs to enhance the dopaminergic (explicit memory) or serotonergic (implicit memory) systems with care for possible negative consequences. For example, a study investigating the link between chronic stress and PTSD found that stress enables a serotonergic memory consolidation process that was not present in unstressed animal subjects (Baratta et al., 2016). The results of this study showed that chronic stress causes proliferation of 5-HT2C receptors in the amygdala that bind to serotonin, thereby creating a heightened sensitivity to serotonin and stronger memory consolidation. This finding suggests that antidepressants such as Prozac and other selective serotonin reuptake inhibitors (SSRIs), when given to recently traumatized individuals, may actually promote stronger traumatic memories (Trafton, 2015).

In ageing and memory loss there may be a compromise in the cAMP process. Kandel (2012) suggests there are two ways to boost memory—either increase the dopaminergic input in the case of explicit memory systems, or slow down the degradation of cAMP by introducing a drug (e.g., Rolipram) that inhibits phosphodiesterase, which would normally break down cAMP. For example, Alzheimer's disease activates inhibitory constraints on the cAMP cycle, and in experiments with mice it has been found that Rolipram restores learning. In the case of Alzheimer's, however, other strategies are available that aim to reduce the toxicity of beta-amyloid to nerve cells (beta-amyloid is the main component of toxic plaques that are believed to play a central role in the development of Alzheimer's disease), rather than boosting the cAMP system (Kandel, 2012).

The Hippocampus

Any discussion of memory, especially explicit memory, would be incomplete without a consideration of the hippocampus. The hippocampi are structures in both hemispheres of the brain, at the base of the temporal lobes, that are likened to the shape of two seahorses—hence their name (from the Greek *hippos*, "horse"). They encode explicit memory, such as the conscious learning of facts taught at school, as well as spatial information, and help to make sense of new information based on previously learned information (Cozolino, 2013). Each hippocampus has slightly different functions: damage to the left hippocampus is associated with difficulties

memory. Yet H.M. could engage in tasks that required practise to improve, such as drawing a figure from its reflection in a mirror, and his ability on the task did improve: he was able to learn the motor coordination skills required to do the task well. This means he could still consolidate implicit memory, but he could not recall actually practising the task—an explicit memory.

Concerning its function in memory, Robert Moss (2016) describes the hippocampus not as a *storage* device but rather an *association* device, because of its role in bringing together various elements stored in the cortex into a coherent and meaningful recall. He conceives discrete bits of information (learning) as stored in cor-

Memory works better when there is context, and the hippocampus puts things in context when encoding and reassembling memory.

in forming new verbal memories, while damage to the right hippocampus produces deficits in other forms of nonverbal memory (Moss, 2016). Memory works better when there is context, and the hippocampus (considered as a whole) puts things in context when encoding and reassembling memory. The hippocampus is active when we navigate space or recollect personal events, and it negotiates the large overlap of spatial/navigational and autobiographical information needed to give us orientation. There are even cells in the hippocampus named "place cells" (O'Keefe & Dostrovsky, 1971) that respond to a certain spatial location to help orient us.

One subject who has famously contributed an enormous amount to our understanding of memory and the role of the hippocampus is a patient named Henry Molaison, commonly known as "H.M.". In 1953, at the age of 27, H.M. had the medial portions of his temporal lobes removed to treat epilepsy. Following this bilateral medial temporal lobectomy, which included most of the hippocampus, H.M.'s seizures were all but eliminated; he seemed to have normal perceptual and motor abilities, and his intelligence actually increased (Pinel & Barnes, 2014). However, the surgery had devastating amnesic effects: H.M. had a memory for events long predating surgery, some retrograde amnesia for events up to two years prior to surgery, but a total inability to form new long-term explicit memories. After surgery he could not remember people, places, events, or experiences for longer than his working memory would allow. The lesson learned from H.M. was that the medial temporal lobes (including the hippocampus) play a critical role in memory, specifically in storing and recalling long-term

tical columns: when we need various bits of information to recreate a memory, cells in the hippocampus are activated and, through the thalamus, connect to various cortical columns to activate those bits of memory simultaneously. Thus, the hippocampus does not itself hold the bits that recreate the memory; instead it coordinates the synchronized activation of those bits held in the cortex. He offers the following example to illustrate:

Quiroga et al. (2005) described a cell in a patient's hippocampus that consistently activated each time different pictures of Jennifer Aniston were shown, but the same cell did not show such activation to other pictures of objects or animals, or other famous

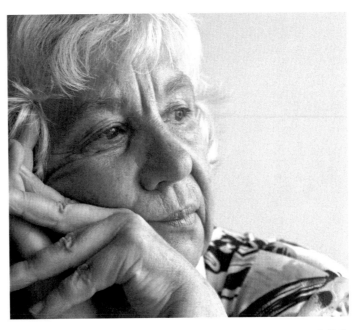

faces. This gives the impression that the cell is the location of the memory. However, my belief is that the visual facial recognition of Jennifer Aniston and the associated word columns of her name occur in separate cortical circuits. For those circuits to be consolidated as an association memory (i.e., her name with her face), the single hippocampal neuron is needed to reactivate the separate circuit columns and the common column in the perirhinal cortex. When shown her picture, the visual column tied to her face activated the common column that in turn activated the hippocampal cell. This explanation fits well with the finding that patients with anterograde amnesia caused by hippocampal damage retain long-term memories that occurred years before they developed the amnesia. Thus, if you know Jennifer Aniston by sight and have future damage resulting in the loss of the hippocampal cell that was involved, you will have no problem recognizing her face and giving her name provided the cortical columns in the circuits relating to her remain intact. (Moss, 2016, p. 18)

Establishing long-term memories that are capable of recall without hippocampal intervention may be possible through the association of circuits between the critical cortical bits—integrative connections of colour, sound, emotion, spatial information, and other bits that are all stimulated at the same time upon recall.

Eleanor Maguire, Professor of Cognitive Neuroscience at University College London, has been exploring with colleagues the way the hippocampus encodes and recreates memory. One of the interesting questions posed by Maguire (2008) was, "Can patients with hippocampal damage and amnesia imagine fictitious experiences?" Similar brain areas are activated in both the imagining of a fictitious experience and the recall of a real episodic memory: we draw on what we know to imagine what we have not experienced. Maguire describes a study of people with hippocampal damage who, when asked to imagine a scene, were unable to do so effectively. They could come up with some of the elements but could not construct a vivid and coherent scene. It was the spatial connectedness of the scene that was wanting in these subjects: there was discontinuity and little ability to create a spatial backdrop in their imagination. Due to the damage in the region, the normal contribution of the hippocampus in recalling various elements and holding them together in context was not available to them.

The concept that consolidation of memories progresses from short-term to long-term has been challenged in a recent study in *Science* suggesting that short-term memory in the hippocampus and long-term consolidation in the cortex form simultaneously (Kitamura et al., 2017). The researchers proposed that the simultaneously formed long-term memories remain "silent" initially but gradually mature, changing in anatomy and physiological activity, until the long-term cortical memory is fully recallable. Using mice and a technique called optogenetics, whereby target cells can be turned on or off with light, the researchers mapped the development of a fear memory. After just one day, memory of the fear event was detected in the cortex. This finding is contrary to the standard theory of memory consolidation (that memories transfer gradually over time), because the memory had already

In the case of childhood traumatic events, it has often been observed that explicit memories are difficult to recall, while implicit emotional memories flood the PTSD sufferer—until there is a change of context in the individual's life, potentially years later, that triggers an explicit recall of the event. However, as Dan Siegel (2012) has noted, delayed recall of explicit autobiographical memory is subject to (unintentional) creative licence:

Recounting the elements of explicit autobiographical memory is a social experience that is profoundly influenced by social interaction.

formed. According to this study, memories are formed rapidly and simultaneously in the prefrontal cortex and the hippocampus: "They're formed in parallel but then they go different ways from there. The prefrontal cortex becomes stronger and the hippocampus becomes weaker," said Mark Morrissey, a co-author on the paper (Trafton, 2017, para. 18). This finding, if supported, will add greatly to our understanding of the functioning of the brain and memory formation.

Recall and Trauma

State-dependent recall describes a phenomenon where our current internal state, if it replicates that at the time a significant event was encoded, can set in motion a spontaneous recall of that memory. A traumatized individual may have the memory of trauma come flooding back when he or she experiences increased heart rate, breathing, or emotion that closely resembles the original response to trauma. In fact, just about anything that matches the original internal experience can trigger some aspect of what the individual went through emotionally and physiologically at the time. Even body posture may be a catalyst for state-dependent recall:

Feedback from postural proprioceptive nerves could have the same memory power as the proprioceptive nerves of internal sensations that must be involved in state-dependent recall under the influence of drugs or alcohol. Asking a client to reconstruct his posture before and during a trauma will often bring details to awareness. However, such a technique must be used with caution, as it can easily stimulate more recall than the client is prepared to handle. Postural state-dependent recall can also be caused unwittingly, as, for example, when a physically abused child either freezes or screams when casually or inadvertently tossed over another's knee in play. (Rothschild, 2000)

Although delayed recollection may be quite accurate, explicit memory is exquisitely sensitive to the conditions of recall. Recounting the elements of explicit autobiographical memory is a social experience that is profoundly influenced by social interaction. Thus what is recounted is not the same as what is initially remembered, and it is not necessarily completely accurate in detail. . . . actual events can be forgotten, and non-experienced "recollections" can be deeply felt to be true memories. (p. 80)

Our minds can be extremely suggestible, and every act of retrieving a memory can be altered by social context and new information. We can be convinced a memory is totally accurate when in fact it may be quite different from its original consolidation (which itself may not have been a completely accurate representation of what really occurred). As psychotherapists, we must be careful to assume a neutral stance with respect to the accuracy of our client's memories: excessive interest in the trauma over the person may generate unconscious pressure on the patient to keep the therapist engaged by elaborating the narrative of trauma" (Siegel, 2012).

Memory Reconsolidation

Memory reconsolidation is a process in which a memory is modified at the level of its neural encoding. It is a substantive change brought about by new learning. The concept of reconsolidation is based on the understanding that when a memory is retrieved from long-term storage, it is held in a labile (unstable) state in short-term memory while it is being utilized (Nader & Hardt, 2009). This process may be a way in which new information is integrated into an existing memory trace—a kind of maintenance of consolidation intended to keep retrieved memory up to date. Most of the laboratory research on reconsolidation has focused on fear conditioning, which psychotherapists have been able to apply to emotional memory.

The work of Bruce Ecker and colleagues (Ecker, Ticic, & Hulley, 2012) has demonstrated that emotional memories can be strengthened, weakened, altered in their details, or completely nullified and cancelled through a reconsolidation process—thereby bringing about a true unlearning of an emotional memory. Reconsolidation is a natural, neural process that can transform an acquired behaviour or emotional response by fundamentally revising the memory associated with it (Ecker, 2015).

It is implicit memory that is mostly involved here, in the form of emotional learning, such as how to avoid particular vulnerabilities and sufferings. These memories, or learnings, are often attained without awareness, entirely within the implicit learning system, in the presence of strong emotions. Accordingly, they can prove powerful and durable. All sorts of emotional and traumatic experiences form implicit emotional learnings whose purpose is essentially adaptive—to help us cope with life as we perceive it. But they frequently become maladaptive later in life when we no longer need to respond in the same self-protective patterns. The child who needs to do outstanding work to attain her parents' love and approval may carry that learning into adult life and become a workaholic, not realizing that her behaviour is more a desperate attempt to meet a ba-

sic emotional need than a reflection of her passion for work. The very behaviour that helped her adapt to circumstances as a child now alienates the people she most wants love and affection from. There is no conscious realization that this is the case: it is implicit, an automation. Such encoding is mainly in the subcortical regions that store implicit, tacit, emotionally urgent, procedural knowledge, rather than the neocortical regions involved in explicit memory, which store conscious, episodic, autobiographical, declarative knowledge (Ecker, 2015).

For psychotherapists, an understanding of memory reconsolidation can be a useful guide to facilitating lasting change in therapy. The ability to identify the mental schemata that underpin unwanted behaviours and to bring them into conscious awareness is a vital step toward transformative change. It works on the principle of consistency: the brain tries to resolve incompatible thought patterns. Rendering a schema of implicit emotional logic explicit, then juxtaposing it with a directly contrasting experience in the conscious perception of client, can cause the original learning to become unstable, providing a unique window for modification. The technique should not be confused with the attempt to construct a new schema in addition to the old, with the two existing in competition. Rather, transformation takes place when the original learning is completely modified at the neural level, so that the physical connections of the original logic no longer exist, but are replaced with a new logic.

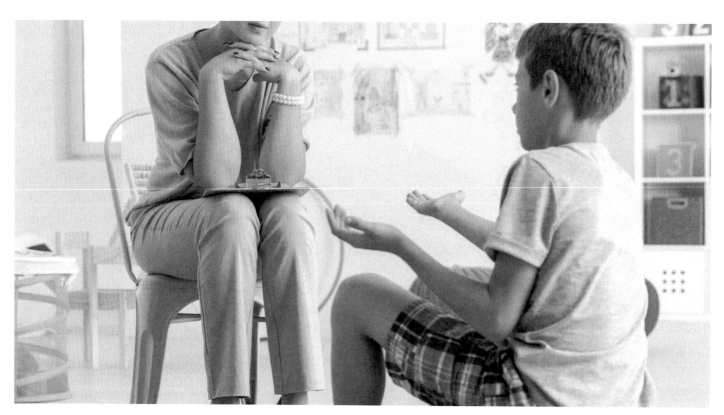

Where are negative emotional memories stored?

Robert Moss, a long-term researcher of human memory and its applications in psychotherapy (Moss, 2006, 2007, 2014; Moss & Mahan, 2014; Moss & Moss, 2014 a, 2014 b), believes that all relevant emotional sensory memories are stored in the cerebral cortex, in the same location where they are originally processed. He further postulates that whenever a new sensory memory is formed in the posterior cortical lobes (i.e., parietal, occipital, and/or temporal), there is a corresponding action memory formed in the frontal cortex. Cortical memories that were formed with significant emotional arousal can in turn reactivate subcortical structures that lead to increased emotional arousal. With this understanding, Moss explains that when subcortical areas (e.g., the amygdala) are activated, it does not mean the memories are stored subcortically (as mentioned above). Moss uses this theory of emotional memory storage to understand how negative emotional memories can affect one's current functioning, as well as one's "personality." He believes these concepts provide support for the argument that psychotherapy can be the most effective way to address such memories. Significantly, his view is that psychotropic medications impact the subcortical level and cannot change the cortical memories once those memories are permanently consolidated.

Moss and colleagues have argued that whenever significant sensory emotional memories are activated in the posterior cortical areas, the projections from the cortex to the lateral amygdala lead to output from the central amygdala. The central amygdala output then leads to quick-onset "fight or flight" patterns such as occur in a panic attack (via projections to the intermediolateral cells in the spinal cord that in turn activate the sympathetic ganglia), but also to prolonged, slower hypothalamic–pituitary–adrenal (HPA) axis effects (via activation of the periventricular nucleus of the hypothalamus). Put simply, the subcortical activation and its associated physical reactions are viewed to result from the activation of sensory negative emotional memories in the cortex.

A point Moss has stressed is that the most influential negative emotional memories are typically housed in the right posterior cortex. Non-verbal emotional processing, including that tied to influential interpersonal relationships, occurs in the right cortex. In his papers, Moss provides detailed support for the argument that the right cortex's design allows faster, less detailed processing. When we communicate non-verbally with one another, it typically involves vocal inflections and facial expressions that lack much detail. The right hemisphere is capable of processing these aspects quickly and accurately. In contrast, the left frontal operculum (the area in and around Broca's area) is where all "verbal" thinking (what is often referred to as "consciousness") occurs. Moss and colleagues have lent further support to the view that this is the home of our internal verbal dialogue. It does not have any direct connections via interhemispheric tracts to the right posterior cortex. Thus, there is no manner to allow direct verbal "conscious" control of the right-hemisphere emotional memories that lead to negative emotional states (e.g., anxiety, dysphoric mood).

One other fascinating idea arising from this research is that in the same manner the left cortex allows us to learn and remember our native *verbal* language, the right hemisphere allows us to learn and remember our native *emotional* language. Both involve the lateral cortex, and both are employed extensively in interpersonal relationships.

PSYCHOLOGICAL NEEDS

Now that we have explored some of the basics of the brain, it is important to put this "wetware" in context with the basic principles of mental functioning. To understand the broader mental functions from the standpoint of their neural underpinnings gives the psychotherapist a sophisticated appreciation of a client's struggles. It also crucially sheds light on why certain therapeutic techniques work and why others may not work so well in any given circumstance. The meta-framework known as neuropsychotherapy represents a multidisciplinary perspective that equips the psychotherapist with a mature understanding across the spectrum from basic neural communication and networks to psychological needs and how we go about enhancing and protecting them. This final section brings together the elements into a bigger picture that I hope will serve you well in clinical practice and inspire you to learn more.

Klaus Grawe developed a view of mental functioning that combined insights from mainstream contemporary psychology with an understanding that "the goals a person forms during his or her life ultimately serve the satisfaction of distinct basic needs" (Grawe, 2007, p.

169). Influenced by Seymour Epstein's cognitive-experiential self-theory (Epstein, 1973, 1980, 1991 1993, 1994, 1998; Teglasi & Epstein, 1998), Grawe defined four key psychological needs that provide the motivation for behaviour: the need for attachment, the need for control/orientation, the need for pleasure/avoidance of pain, and the need for self-enhancement (Grawe, 2007; see also Epstein, 1994, p. 715 for the origins of these four needs). Implicit motivational schemas, which we will discuss below, are designed to satisfy these four psychological needs via either approach-driven (primarily cortical processes) or avoidance-driven (primarily limbic processes) behaviour in what Epstein describes as an emotionally driven experiential system (Epstein, 1994). Here we explore these basic psychological needs:

Motivational Schemas

A motivational schema is, at root, a neural network developed to satisfy and protect basic needs. Schemas can be broadly divided into two classes: approach schemata and avoidance schemata (see figure below). Approach and avoidance schemata operate on different

BASIC NEEDS AND MOTIVATIONAL SCHEMAS

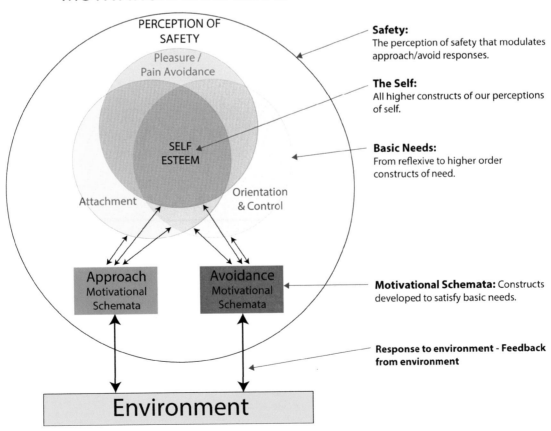

Safety: The perception of safety that modulates approach/avoid responses.

The Self: All higher constructs of our perceptions of self.

Basic Needs: From reflexive to higher order constructs of need.

Motivational Schemata: Constructs developed to satisfy basic needs.

Response to environment - Feedback from environment

neural pathways (Grawe, 2007). If an individual grows up in an environment where needs have been met, especially during the critical early attachment phase, then approach schemas of interacting with the environment are likely to develop, resulting in approach-oriented behaviour. Conversely, an individual whose needs are continually threatened and violated is likely to develop avoidance schemas that will motivate insecure, anxious, and avoidant behaviour. Bowlby's (1973, 1988) attachment theory furnishes a critical understanding of the foundation of mental schemata, explaining how securely attached children develop primarily approach motivational schemas and insecurely attached children develop avoidance motivational schemas.

Approach and avoidance motivation has a long history. The concept first appeared in the writings of Greek philosopher Democritus of Abdera (460–370 B.C.E.), broadly seeking to explain behaviour as directed either toward positive stimuli or away from negative stimuli (Elliot, 2008). The full spectrum of approach–avoidance motivation includes such orienting exteroceptive reflexes as the startle response, salivary reflex, and pain withdrawal. But for the purposes of neuropsychotherapy, approach and avoidance schemata are psychological orientations toward or away from stimuli (whether concrete objects, events, and possibilities or abstract subjective representations) that may or may not have a corresponding somatic movement or action. Furthermore, "movement toward" can represent either *gaining* something positive that is currently absent or *keeping* something positive that is currently present (in functional terms, "continuing toward"). Likewise, "movement away" can represent either *getting away* from something negative that is currently present or *keeping away* from something negative that is currently absent (in functional terms, "continuing away from"; Elliot, 2008, p. 8).

The consistency theory model conceptualizes all behaviour as the product of approach and avoidance motivations. The somewhat binary nature of this view may appear over-simplistic at first glance, but its complexity lies in the fact that many approach and avoidance schemata can be operating in parallel (as in the case of motivational discordance; Grawe, 2007) and in a hierarchical manner (Elliot, 2006), to service not only our basic psychological needs but also physiological reflexes as we navigate our experiences of the world.

For the psychotherapist, there is clarity in understanding it is the motivational schemata that are the cause of distress and, consequently, the target for change. These schemata are developed through right-lateralized implicit emotional learning during attachment and are represented by physical neural networks. The networks can be changed, quite literally, in a therapeutic setting by intersubjective right brain-to-right brain regulation that uses controlled incongruence to achieve memory reconsolidation, thereby transforming existing neural networks.

According to consistency theory, there are three ways the mental system can experience inconsistency: through *approach incongruence, avoidance incongruence* and *discordance*. These upset the neural harmony of the system, creating a system demand to reduce such stress or dissonance.

Approach incongruence. If an individual tends towards avoidance motivational schemas—that is, if there is an established neural propensity to avoid perceived threats to basic needs rather than seek to satisfy those needs—he or she can experience incongruent signals due to unfulfilled approach schemas. To illustrate, consider a young woman who has a desire to meet a man, but fear of rejection prevents her from placing herself in situations where she may meet a potential partner. The avoidant motivational schema is well established to protect her from the pain of rejection by another human being, and prioritizes the maintenance of whatever self-esteem and control over circumstances she has. However, there is at the same time a desire represented in another motivational schema to approach, to apprehend, to secure a loving relationship with a partner and satisfy the need for attachment. It is when this latter desire is suppressed or overridden by the stronger avoidance schema that the individual experiences approach incongruence.

Avoidance incongruence. When attempts at avoidance ultimately fail, and what was feared actually happens, the individual experiences avoidance incongruence. To continue the previous illustration, if the young woman does go to a local dance to meet a potential partner and is, after all, rejected, she will experience avoidance incongruence—the very undesired consequences her avoidance schema had motivated her to protect herself from.

Discordance. Discordance occurs when two or more motivational schemas are activated simultaneously and are incompatible with one another. This is not an incongruence between perception and goal but rather two incompatible goals being activated simultaneously.

Incongruence and discordance, and the affect that accompanies them, can occur implicitly or explicitly and create inconsistency in the system. Continual inconsist-

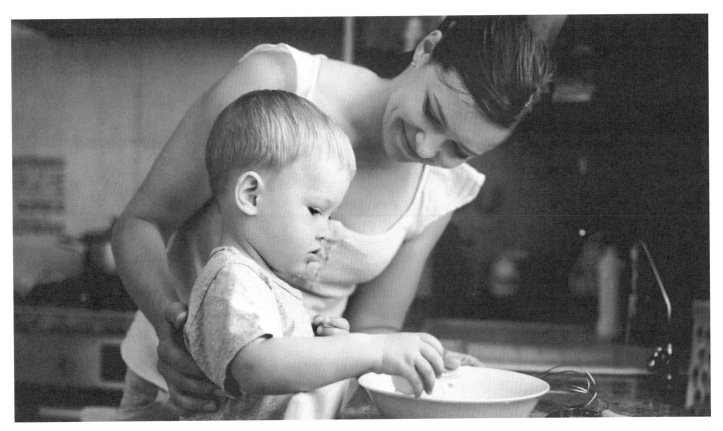

ency can impair an individual's effective engagement with the environment and lead to increasingly avoidant tendencies, stress, negative emotions, anxiety, and a range of serious mental difficulties, as limbic survival mechanisms dominate to protect the individual who is descending into a highly complex state of stress.

The consistency model conceptualizes behaviour as an attempt to attain or protect the object of basic needs through motivational schemas that have been shaped by earlier experiences (in particular of attachment), in a way that provides agreement with the individual's perception of the world and internal model of the world and him or herself.

There are current attempts to refine Grawe's model so that the basic psychological needs are portrayed in a less linear fashion and are seen as overlapping in their neural arrangement, with the superimposition of the basic needs yielding a higher-order construct of "self". The figure below shows a refinement by Rossouw (2014) in which the higher-order construct of "self" emerges from the neural milieu of needs and motivational schemata.

Attachment

John Bowlby (1973, 1988) demonstrated convincingly that the basic need of an infant is the physical proximity of a primary attachment figure, ushering the importance of attachment into mainstream psychology. Bowlby (1973) articulated the basis of his attachment theory in three central postulates that could be summarized this way:

- A child with an available, trusted caregiver will be less anxious than one without such a caregiver.

- Trust or lack of trust in the availability of the caregiver will translate into a similar expectancy of relationships later in life.

- The expectations a child has of a caregiver are relatively true of the actual experiences of the caregiver.

Bowlby referred to this theory of attachment as the internal working model, a concept taken from Kenneth Craik, who proposed that an organism carries a "small-scale model" of external reality in its head (Wallin, 2007, p. 26). In essence, early dyadic relationships, especially with primary caregivers, form implicit memories from which a child constructs schemas, or ways of understanding and interacting with the world. A parent's approach to his or her infant shapes the very structure of its developing brain through

Integrated Model of the Base Elements of the Theory of Neuropsychotherapy (Rossouw, 2014, p. 57)

proximity and gaze (Schore, 2012). As therapist and interpersonal neurobiology instructor Bonnie Badenoch has put it, "What is alight in the parental brain lights up in the newborn brain. It is as though the parent is passing on the family's emotional legacy in regards to relationships through these initial firings and wirings" (Badenoch, 2008, p. 53).

Mary Ainsworth, a colleague of Bowlby, developed an empirical method for assessing attachment in infants called the Strange Situation Protocol, based on Bowlby's attachment theory (Ainsworth, Blehar, Waters, & Wall, 1978). Ainsworth observed the behaviour patterns of young children when they were separated and then reunited with their mothers in a controlled environment. Several attachment styles were identified at this point: secure attachment, insecure-avoidant attachment, and insecure-ambivalent attachment (Ainsworth et al., 1978; Badenoch, 2008). Later, Mary Main and colleagues (Main & Solomon, 1986) identified another style they called insecure-disorganized/disorientated attachment.

Unsurprisingly, the children who were found to thrive in life were those who had formed secure, rather than insecure, attachment patterns. Attachment patterns start to form in the first months of life—a time when brain development is extremely rapid, the sympathetic nervous system is dominant, and right-hemisphere limbic learning is critical (Badenoch, 2008)—and they lay the foundation for the motivational schemas that ultimately drive behaviour.

Orientation and Control

Epstein (1990) characterized the need for orientation and control as the most fundamental of all human needs. According to Powers' (1973) perceptual control theory, this need plays out in a pervasive striving for perceptions of reality that are consistent with the individual's goals, and this striving is a major driver of behaviour and mental life. If we want to be respected or to be financially secure, we will act towards achieving a sense that we are. To attain such a goal requires control over our environment, or at least our perception of the environment. Grawe (2007) added that control was not only about manipulating or regulating the environment or relationships to achieve goals, but also about maximizing the number of options we are free to act upon. How we then choose to take up the options available to us will be determined by our motivational schemas.

A sense of control begins in infancy, in the context of attachment, with the child having the volition to manipulate the environment to meet his or her needs. An infant crying when hungry has the desired outcome of summoning Mother who has food. If the child cries for food and no food comes, there is an incongruence (the gap between what the child needs and what she perceives she has), and with such a violation of the need for attachment there is a corresponding violation of the need for control. A satisfaction of the need for control, on the other hand, causes a reduction in distress, which in turn strengthens the sense of control.

There is a component, or an understanding, of control that can be described as the need for orientation—that is, to have an accurate appraisal of a situation, and to understand what is going on. To gain such clarity about one's situation, and what can be done to improve it, is an important aspect of control. It is a common experience in psychotherapy to see a better sense of control gained simply through understanding a situation with greater clarity. In view of this need for orientation, effective (disorder-specific and problem-specific) therapeutic interventions are always accompanied by a more optimal satisfaction of the need for control.

Pleasure Maximization and Pain Minimization

Freud, in his theory of personality, postulated a single fundamental need that he characterized as the pleasure principle: the need to maximize pleasure and minimize pain (Freud 1920/1959). Epstein (1994) considered this a core need, as did Grawe (2007).

The basic premise of this need is that we are moti-

The prefrontal cortex (PFC) is the most underdeveloped region of the brain at birth, and its architecture is developed in response to our experiences as we grow. It is highly adaptive, shaping the way we see ourselves and the world as we experience life. The capacity of the PFC to regulate emotions by inhibiting sympathetically driven, survival-oriented neural networks while increasing calming parasympathetic vagal activity is dependent on its early development. Experiences of abuse, neglect, and trauma typically result in a PFC less capable of emotional self-regulation. Conversely, experiences of caregivers who sensitively help navigate emotions, soothe, and demonstrate self-regulation—essentially creating emotional safety—foster the development of a PFC capable of regulating the limbic system and providing a flexible sympathetic/parasympathetic balance.

Psychotherapy is an opportunity for a less well developed PFC to gain the skills of emotional self-regulation that may not have been instilled in childhood. This kind of therapy is literally about rewiring the brain so that the PFC has stronger mechanisms of control over the fear-driven emotional brain areas like the amygdala, and can apply the parasympathetic "brake" more readily and flexibly via the vagus nerve to the heart, increasing heart-rate variability (we will discuss heart-rate variability in a later section). Psychotherapy can help us be more aware of our habitual anticipation of threat and to choose new experiences that make us feel safer and more flexible in our responses. In short, we can choose to change the heart–mind connection (Peckham, 2015).

vated to attain pleasant experiences or states and avoid unpleasant or painful ones. These states may be physical, psychological, emotional, or social. Neurologically there is an automatic, implicit evaluation of experience as either "good" or "bad", to the degree that there is a continual monitoring of our experiences (one aspect of this process is known as feedback-related negativity; see Hajcak, Moser, Holroyd, & Simons, 2006; Nieuwenhuis, Slagter, Von Geusau, Heslenfeld, & Holroyd, 2005). Humans have a motivation to maximize experiences of the good and limit the bad, even in the case of suffering "for the greater good"—the denial of some pleasures to attain something of greater worth. What constitutes "good", "pleasurable", "beautiful", and the like is dependent upon the individual and how his or her experience is consistent with the satisfaction of the other basic needs. Grawe contends that the individual is in a maximal state when his or her "current perceptions and goals are completely congruent with one another, and the transpiring mental activity is not disturbed by any competing intentions" (2007, p. 244). This maximal state—a state of pleasure—is comparable to Mihaly Csikszentmihalyi's (1991) concept of "flow", which describes our intrinsic motivation to align our perception of experience with our intentions.

Just how a person will size up the world around him is dependent on both his prior experience and his momentary state. For example, a hot drink on a very hot day may be evaluated more negatively than an ice-cold drink, and vice versa on a cold day; this is a state-dependent evaluation. By contrast, the experience of going on a roller-coaster is likely to be far less state-dependent—one individual may evaluate it as bad and another as good, according to each person's prior experience with roller-coasters. The relearning of taste preferences is a complex process influenced by motives such as social compliance and positive self-evaluations, yet the same automatic evaluative process is in play. The development of a taste for wine, for example, may be motivated by a need for social acceptance (attachment and self-esteem), but ultimately becomes an automatic preference for wine as part of the neural evaluative process.

When a situation is evaluated either positively or negatively, it triggers an approach or avoidance tendency, meaning that our mental activity is primed in a certain direction. For example, someone who evaluates New York cab drivers as bad on the basis of past negative experiences may be primed to "jump" at the sudden lane changes made by the driver. Another person with a more positive evaluation of New York cab drivers may not be startled or fearful at all at the same sudden lane changes. This motivational priming is essentially an orientation of the motivational system toward either approach or avoidance behaviour in response to certain cues in our environment.

Mental processes transpire more easily and quickly when the good/bad evaluation is compatible or synchronized with the behavioural approach–avoidance orientation. In other words, when evaluations and behavioural orientations are consistent, the mental system works more efficiently and with less stress.

Self-Esteem Enhancement

The need for self-enhancement or self-esteem has been called the "master sentiment" (McDougall, 1936, p. 224) and "the basic law of human life" (Becker, 1971, p. 66). It is the only one of the four needs that is distinctly human. Self-esteem has been defined as "an individual's subjective evaluation of her or his worth as a person. If a person believes that she is a person of worth and value, then she has high self-esteem, regardless of whether her self-evaluation is validated by others or corroborated by external criteria" (Trzesniewski, Donnellan, & Robins,

2013, p. 60). However, there has been debate over the importance of this construct, with some arguing that self-esteem is essential (Orth, Robins, & Widaman, 2012) and others considering it of limited value in that it is likely a reflection of other processes (Boden, Fergusson, & Horwood, 2008, Zeigler-Hill, 2013). The self-esteem that Grawe conceptualized as a basic need is a global one that is secure and congruent as opposed to unstable, narcissistic, or discrepant (see Park & Crocker, 2013). Nevertheless, it is possible that self-esteem is a complex construction emerging from more fundamental needs—an outcome of self-perception, and indeed of a perception that may be culturally driven and fail to qualify as a basic need (Dahlitz & Rossouw, 2014).

In some cases, to preserve the greatest number of needs, one need may be "sacrificed". For example, the maintenance of low self-esteem may be an avoidance pattern utilized to fulfil another need such as preventing pain or preventing loss of control, or to protect existing self-esteem from further degradation. Alternatively, avoidance of high self-esteem may win the individual acceptance, thus meeting a need for attachment—which, in a roundabout way, satisfies some aspect of self-esteem. In these scenarios the tendency to self-esteem enhancement can be regarded as part of the approach system, and self-esteem protection can be regarded as part of the avoidance system. The exact reasons for an individual maintaining low self-esteem may be complex, but in context with other needs, it is safe to assume this is a compromise aimed at achieving overall need fulfilment/protection as best the individual can.

Those who do satisfy the need for enhanced self-esteem are characterized by better mental health. These individuals will take opportunities to enhance their self-esteem through approach motivational schemas. They will evaluate themselves more positively than objective observers—in fact it has been found that an unrealistically positive perception of self satisfies the self-esteem enhancement need and is itself a good indicator of overall mental health. Mentally healthy individuals also have a skewed perception of their place in social context, often seeing themselves as "above average" within the general population. Indeed, striving for an absolutely realistic self-evaluation may not be in their best interests for mental well-being. Deluding oneself in the meeting of basic needs can lead to positive feelings and in turn to attaining a better state, a bit like a self-fulfilling prophecy. Depressed individuals, however, who have a more pessimistic view of reality, do not share this delusion and are prone to further mental problems.

Operating out of avoidance schemas, these individuals experience life, and take on roles, in a way often detrimental to self-esteem.

Approach/Avoid Networks

A view of mental function based on the binary notion of approach and avoidance motivational systems can prove useful. We are either "approaching" to apprehend something, or we are "avoiding" to preserve and protect. Such approach/avoid systems operate independently of one another and have independent neural substrates and mechanisms (Grawe, 2007). They can be activated in a parallel fashion, although equally strong systems will tend to mutually inhibit each other. As we have learnt earlier, there are significant differences between the left and right hemispheres of the brain, and these are reflected in approach/avoidance motivations such that the left hemisphere is biased toward approach (positive) emotions and the right toward avoidance (negative) emotions (Canli, Desmond, Zhao, Glover & Gabrieli, 1998; Davidson 1992; Paradiso et al., 1999). It is possible to conceive of behaviour as an outcome based on the summation of approach/avoid calculations in our conscious and unconscious mind. This is an im-

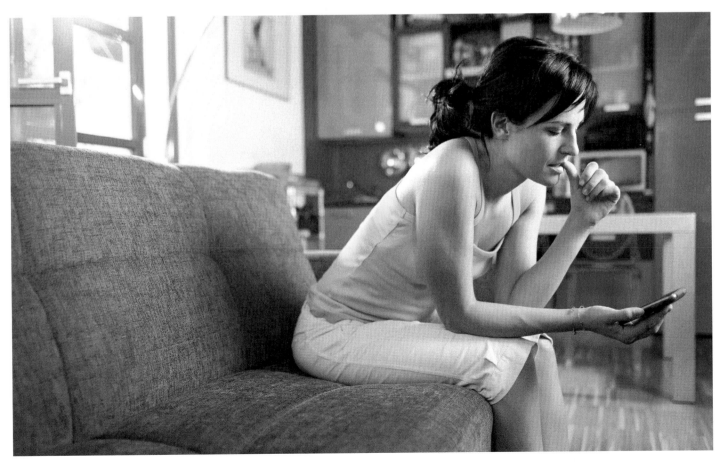

portant concept to come to grips with.

Basic needs have a neural foundation from birth that initiates behaviour like crying, sucking, and wiggling the body to meet those needs (Panksepp & Biven, 2012). These genetically governed behaviours are the beginning of what will develop into much more personal and sophisticated motivational goals. The first need that develops into an "approach" goal is the need for proximity of the primary attachment figure. As the infant experiences encounters with its mother, it starts to develop a repertoire of behaviours to influence the mother to meet her needs. Neural activation patterns emerge that represent this and other goals, and these are strengthened with the help of oxytocin and do-

pamine. Both baby and mother are rewarded by oxytocin and dopamine release when in loving, mutually satisfying connectedness. The increasing strength and complexity of these neural patterns continues to form circuits, which are readily activated, leading eventually to very sophisticated and spontaneously activated schemas. The specific groups of motivational schemas that develop to satisfy the basic needs of an individual are infinitely richer and more multifaceted than what might be suggested by the classification of just a few attachment styles. As the individual grows, motivational goals are shaped by his or her wider environment along with social expectations, limitations, and other cultural forces, shaping the neural architecture of personal motivational schemas.

On a physiological level, approach goals are associated with the left dorsolateral prefrontal cortex (PFC), while avoidance is more closely aligned with the right. For the processing of emotions, the left ventromedial PFC is associated with positive emotions and the right for negative emotions. These motivations and evaluations of approach/positive and avoidance/negative are thus physiologically lateralized across the brain. There are correlations to this same lateralization in the deeper limbic system, giving credence to the theory that approach and avoidance are indeed neurally independent systems.

As they relate to pleasure maximization (approach) and pain minimization (avoidance), approach and avoidance schemas may seem to be opposites, like a positive and negative charge. But they are just different goals with different modes of operation. The approach schema is about closing the gap between a desired goal and perceived reality to attain that goal which satisfies a need. There is often progress toward a goal, with rewards along the way, culminating in attainment (or otherwise) of that goal. However, the avoidance schema is about increasing the distance between something undesirable and perceived reality, often to preserve or protect a basic need—a goal frequently not achieved, but nonetheless necessitating a state of continuous surveillance. When pursuing a positive goal, like completing a university course, it is relatively easy to determine whether one has come closer to the goal: there are sub-goals and markers (such as completing a semester) along the way to the final destination of the goal. However, avoidance goals require constant control, as well as distributed, rather than focused, attention. For example, a husband may be anxious to avoid an argument with his wife: he has to keep vigilant, watch what he says, be careful to read the signs of a possible argument, and he can never reach the goal of avoidance because there is always the possibility that conflict may come in the future. This sort of avoidance is more a matter of continuous attention, and often anxious tension, than simply apprehending a concrete goal. Individuals with strongly formed avoidance goals (or with a dominance of avoidance over approach goals) experience fewer positive emotions and less satisfaction of need because of the disproportionate amount of energy and focus invested in avoidance. In fact, strongly developed avoidance tendencies, both implicit and explicit, have many unfavourable effects on mental health, self-esteem and general well-being (Grawe, 2007).

How does this translate to therapy? In a nutshell, we should aim to reduce the inclination toward avoidance goals and promote more positive approach goals to satisfy basic needs. The behaviour of depressed clients can frequently be attributed to a hyperactivation of avoidance schemas, which inhibits approach schemas and invites the negative impact of stress hormones that damage the hippocampus and deactivate the anterior cingulate cortex. A therapy that can weaken the established avoidance tendencies and gradually reactivate the approach system will revitalize activity in the anterior cingulate cortex and strengthen PFC connections—concrete developments that will likely result in a positive change for the client.

In the previous section on Memory we learnt that dopamine is a critical factor in establishing new learning and reinforcing neural change. Dopamine is the reinforcing agent and represents neural motivation, or motivational salience, in establishing behaviour. Any behaviour that is reinforced involves the release of dopamine. Because dopamine is essential for motivation and learning (establishing and reinforcing synaptic connections), in therapy, learning must have high motivational salience to be effective. In real terms, without the activation of the dopamine system, substantial, positive long-term learning will not take place. Dopamine is the intrinsic motivator and energizer of approach/avoidance schemas and is therefore of central importance to the therapeutic process.

The Consistency Principle

Consistency is the overarching concept of systemic agreement that can be considered a "core principle of mental functioning" (Grawe, 2007, p. 168). The myriad simultaneously occurring processes in the nervous system function optimally only to the extent that the various elements of the system remain in harmony and are not conflicted. This is a foundational principle of neuropsychotherapy.

The now famous Stroop test (Stroop, 1935) is a classic example of activating conflicting mental processes and thus compromising performance speed as the an-

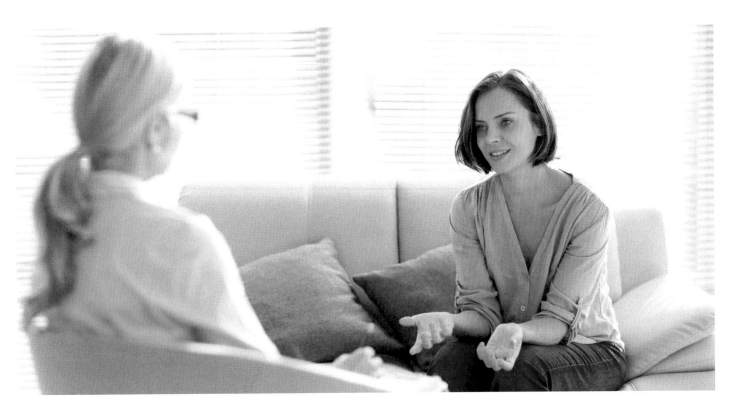

terior cingulate cortex and the dorsolateral PFC work through inconsistent patterns to arrive at a resolution (Milham, 2003). On a more complex level, an individual's experience of the world, internal model of the world, and meeting of needs can be in conflict—a state of internal inconsistency from which dissatisfaction and stress arise. To effect neural, and therefore therapeutic, change, we need to induce a state of controlled incongruence within a system striving for consistency.

The consistency theory (Grawe, 2004, 2007) view of mental functioning is derived both from broadly accepted findings that goals and schemas govern mental activity and from Grawe's own argument that goal formation is developed to satisfy four basic psychological needs: attachment, orientation & control, avoidance of pain/maximization of pleasure, and self-esteem enhancement. The core constructs of consistency and congruence are the keys to understanding the development and maintenance of both normal and pathological mental processes.

Consistency is described as the "compatibility of many simultaneously transpiring mental processes" (Grawe, 2007, p. 170), and is a systemic demand, on a neural level, for harmonious neural flow. When the relationship between intrapsychic processes and states is harmonious, there exists a state of consistency. The human nervous system strives to avoid inconsistency and develops various mechanisms to move from a dissonant, inconsistent state to a more harmonious state. Consistency regulation is predominantly unconscious and only rises to conscious awareness under exceptional circumstances. The mechanisms an individual uses to avoid or correct significant inconsistencies have been termed defence mechanisms, coping strategies, or affect regulation.

Congruence, a construct that comes under the umbrella of consistency, is the harmony or compatibility between motivational goals and current perceptions of reality. According to Powers (1973), incongruence signals are generated from the feedback mechanism that contrasts our perceptions with our goals. Grawe argues that "an elevated incongruence level can be regarded . . . as a highly complex stress state" (Grawe, 2007, p. 172).

Change

A focus on the neural underpinnings of behaviour provides an opportunity in therapy for empathy between client and therapist, because it reduces any stigma or self-blame associated with a pathologizing perspective and allows for better understanding of psychotherapeutic techniques and theory (Grawe, 2007). The clinical application of this knowledge focuses on strengthening clients' resources from the core of their motivational system to facilitate an increasingly robust approach to self and the world (Flückiger, Wüsten, Zinbarg, & Wampold, 2009). Such approach motivation ultimately leads to better need satisfaction and subsequent mental wellbeing. In practice, this entails establishing a "safe" therapeutic alliance to facilitate approach patterns that will satisfy basic needs, down-regulate stress activation, and optimize new, positive neural connections while reinforcing existing ones (Rossouw, 2014).

From a clinical perspective, it is controllable incongruence that becomes the mechanism of change within the therapeutic dyad. To recap, incongruence is the discrepancy between an individual's perception of reality (his or her actual experience) and beliefs, expectations, and goals. Such incongruence will cause inconsistency within the mental system. Controllable incongruence describes a situation of incongruence that the individual believes he or she can cope with—it may be a challenge, but not an overwhelming one. Uncontrollable incongruence, on the other hand, is a circumstance that exceeds one's ability to cope, or at least one's belief in that ability, with the mismatch between what is experienced and one's goals.

Uncontrollable incongruence, then, is a stressful state that heightens arousal potentially beyond one's window of tolerance and, if not resolved, can result in a hyperactivated HPA-axis cascade, releasing damaging amounts of glucocorticoids into the system. In a regulated stress response, a feedback loop will down-regulate the HPA-axis activation and attenuate the release of stress hormones (Kandel, Schwartz, Jessell, Siegelbaum, & Hudspeth, 2012). In a state of continued stress—as with unresolved uncontrollable incongruence—this feedback mechanism is overridden, and a continued

flow of glucocorticoids can inhibit the formation of new synapses (new learning) while degenerating existing glutamate synapses, especially in the hippocampus, destabilizing previously formed neural connections (established learning) and even inducing complex negative structural changes in various brain regions (Lupien, McEwen, Gunnar, & Heim, 2009; Popoli, Yan, McEwen, & Sanacora, 2012). To limit such a destructive cascade of events, the therapist should aim to introduce a sense of control in order to reduce arousal and in turn restore HPA-axis regulation.

Controllable incongruence is a state in which a stressor (the incongruence) is raising arousal levels through sympathetic excitation and noradrenergic activation and may exceed a certain threshold to activate the HPA-axis, but the situation is perceived as manageable, and feedback loops are intact to down-regulate the stress response in a timely manner. Such a controlled stress reaction causes a moderate amount of adrenalin to permeate the nervous system, including the neurons, glia, and endothelial cells, which can facilitate a constructive response to the incongruence in the form of learning. As adrenergic receptors are stimulated at blood vessels and astrocytes, glucose release is increased, with a corresponding increase in metabolism. This metabolic increase, in conjunction with the release of neurotrophic factors from astrocytes (Verkhratsky & Butt, 2007) and the stimulation of adrenergic receptors, will help stabilize neural connections activated when coping with the incongruence (in a process representing existing coping strategies) and also improve the facilitation of new neural connections (new coping strategies)—the opposite to what occurs in the case of uncontrollable incongruence. In fact, rising to the challenge of controlling incongruence is essential to "the formation of ever more complex and differentiated neural circuits to an optimal expression of [one's] genetic potential" (Grawe, 2007, p. 222).

As the individual continues to deal with a controllable incongruent situation, coping behaviour is established. Eventually such situations will no longer elicit a stress response, because the neural networks required to effectively assess and cope with the situation are now firmly in place. This is a key goal of therapy: to strengthen existing coping skills and facilitate new ones on a neurobiological level of resilience. The crucial point is that such learning is not possible, on a neural level, in the overwhelming situation of uncontrollable incongruence, where an overabundance of cortisol is

hampering, even degenerating, synaptic connections. Within the safety of the therapeutic alliance, stress responses can be down-regulated to a state of optimal learning, and incongruence can be broken down into controllable, manageable parts to which new strategies can be applied.

What are the practical steps to therapy? Grawe (2007) points to what he calls motivational priming and resource activation as key elements for a controllable incongruence learning state (see also Flückiger, Caspar, Grosse Holtforth & Willutzki, 2009; Flückiger & Grosse Holtforth, 2008). Motivational priming is the priming of the approach system via positive emotional experiences within the therapy session. Such a strategy focuses on positive need-satisfying experiences that are compatible with the client's goals, particularly at the beginning of the session, to provide some positive satisfaction of orientation/control, attachment, pain avoidance, or self-esteem enhancement needs. Establishing an effective therapeutic alliance is one example of a positive activation of a need (attachment) that would prime the client toward approach-orientated tendencies within the session. Resource activation is the therapist's skill of identifying existing resources, characteristics, and abili-

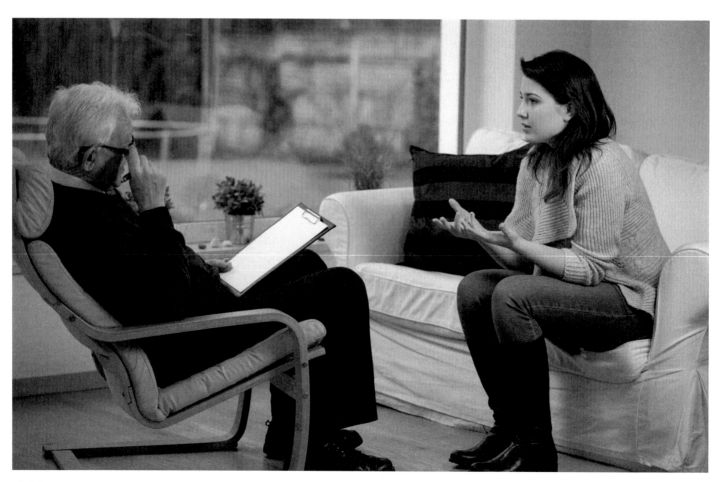

ties of the client that can be positively emphasized during the session in order to enhance the client's feelings of control or self-esteem and increase his or her tolerance for short-term increases in inconsistency during therapy (Smith & Grawe, 2003).

This focus on the client's healthy psychological attributes is in contrast to the problem activation that is stressed in all major therapy schools, yet both play a role in explaining therapeutic change (Gassmann & Grawe, 2006). Flückiger, Wüsten, Zinbarg, and Wampold (2009) noted, "Upon starting therapy or counselling, people seeking help often feel hopeless and have given up believing in their own problem-solving resources. It is therefore the counselor's job to reactivate the experience of that person's self-effectiveness. A counselor should pick up on the person's existing strengths and skills" (p. 2). Ideally, motivational priming and resource activation should be facilitated early in the therapeutic process and emphasized throughout sessions. In this atmosphere of activated resources, therapy has a much greater chance of success (Gassmann & Grawe, 2006).

The importance of a feeling of safety within the therapeutic dyad cannot be overstated. A client must feel safe for therapy to attenuate the destructive stress responses already described and in order to take advantage of controllable incongruence as a mechanism of change. Only from a place of trust and security can an individual actively engage within his or her window of tolerance and take advantage of the brain's natural neuroplasticity. Research has shown that "a safe, enriched environment actually facilitates the development of new neural patterns, which, in turn, leads to enhanced attachment and control, and stress reduction. Psychotherapeutic approaches that provide safe environments will thus enhance the positive social interaction that is an essential element of healthy neural proliferation" (Allison & Rossouw, 2013, p. 23). To establish such a safe environment requires a down-regulation of avoidance motivational schemas that may be activated.

Therapists will appreciate the logic of applying what is essentially a bottom-up approach to deal with the physiological stress response before attempting to facilitate effective neural change and proliferation. The affectively focused right brain-to-right brain therapeutic relationship, mediated via so-called "mirror neuron" activity, can establish safety for a client by down-regulating limbic reactivity and communicating an empathic,

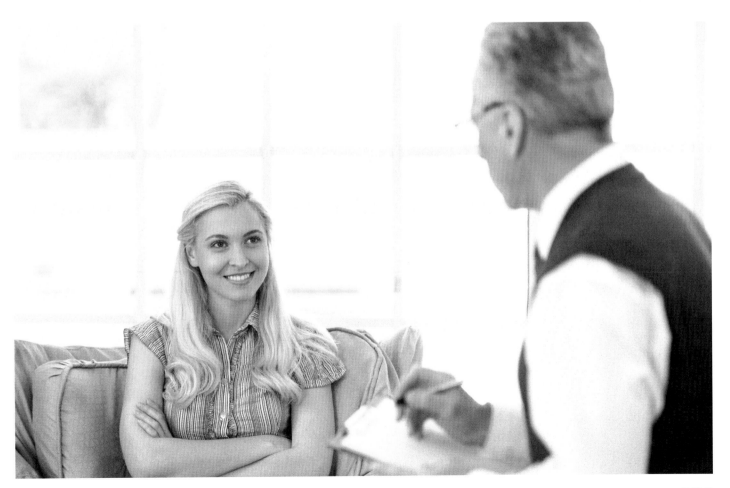

supportive stance that satisfies the basic need for attachment (Schore, 2012). Once a client feels safe, the therapist has created the ideal environment for facilitating neural proliferation in an integrative manner, because the nervous system is essentially socially oriented: it thrives on interpersonal love, acceptance, and security (Cozolino, 2014; Schore, 2012, Siegel, 2012).

Having discussed fear and anxiety in some detail, in turning our attention to therapy it is important to reiterate the practical implications of what happens to a client when anxiety increases—a decrease in cortical blood flow in the left PFC and an increase in the right PFC and limbic system, inhibiting the ability of the left PFC to modulate emotional arousal. When the left PFC is engaged and activated and the limbic system is downregulated, as is our goal in a safe therapeutic environment, more cortical blood flows to the left PFC, and the client can manage his or her emotions more easily. This works in much the same way that a sympathetic response can cause peripheral shut-down to shunt more blood to essential organs like the heart when there is an immediate threat. When a system like the left PFC is required to down-regulate an over-reaction elicited by an overactive amygdala, for example, yet is robbed of the resources needed to do that job (blood flow and the precious oxygen it supplies), then we have a problem: the client is in the grip of a feeling of uncontrollable incongruence.

One of the ways to mitigate the problem of an essential control system like the PFC going "offline" in times of stress is to increase its integrative connectivity to those areas that need higher-order control, such as the amygdala. Mindfulness is one practice that can achieve this. Described as focused attention in the present without judgment (Kabat-Zinn, 1994, 2013), mindfulness can increase mid-PFC and right anterior insula activity and thickening, and increase activity in the superior temporal gyrus and anterior cingulate (Badenoch, 2008). The result is an enhanced integration of these systems with the limbic system, providing better modulatory control over amygdala overreactions and fostering a propensity to approach rather than avoid challenging situations (Siegel, 2012). Such an increase in control brings previously overwhelming situations back into the realm of controllable incongruence. Research suggests that meditative practices like mindfulness not only increase the integration and plasticity of neural networks, but can also offset ageing processes and increase our ability to be present, attuned and compassionate with others (Badenoch, 2008).

Siegel (2007) suggests another "mindful" strategy to gain greater prefrontal management of limbic responsiveness that involves a change in language. Rather than saying, "I'm sad," an example of self-talk that would facilitate a greater sense of separation for the client between the self and the emotion is, "There's a feeling of sadness right now." Positioning the emotion as an objectively observable phenomenon apart from the "observing self" elicits a greater sense of control over what would otherwise be an immersive emotional experience.

Whatever mindful strategy is utilized, there are some common outcomes to such practices: less dysregulation and reactivity to emotional experiences; remaining present with feelings, thoughts, or actions without being distracted; the ability to label beliefs, opinions, emotions, and expectations; and having a nonjudgmental stance toward our experiences (Badenoch, 2008; Baer, Smith, Hopkins, Krietemeyer, & Toney, 2006).

Motivational priming, resource activation, the creation of safety, and techniques like mindfulness are all designed to bring the client into a place of optimal learning where incongruence is perceived to be within the client's window of tolerance, controllable, and therefore an opportunity for new learning and positive change. Seeing positive change and a happier, healthier client is surely the therapist's primary goal. With a neurobiologically informed framework, important practical steps are revealed to seeing our clients' behaviours emerge from the influence of motivational schemata that were developed naturally to preserve or enhance needs. The therapist armed with an understanding of how the brain works and influences the mind can proceed with more awareness and skill than ever before. It is my hope that this book has inspired you to learn more about the human neurobiology for your clients, your practice, and for yourself.

REFERENCES

Aben, B., Stapert, S., & Blokland, A. (2012). About the distinction between working memory and short-term memory. *Frontiers in Psychology, 3*, 301. doi:10.3389/fpsyg.2012.00301

Agerberth, B., & Gudmundsson, G. H. (2006). Host antimicrobial defence peptides in human disease. *Current Topics in Microbiology and Immunology, 306*, 67–90.

Ainsworth, M. D., Blehar, M. C., Waters, E., & Wall, S. (1978). Patterns of attachment: A psychological study of the strange situation. Hillsdale, NJ: Lawrence Erlbaum Associates.

Alexander, G. E., DeLong, M. R., & Strick, P. L. (1986). Parallel organization of functionally segregated circuits linking basal ganglia and cortex. *Annual Review of Neuroscience, 9*, 357–381.

Allison, K. L., & Rossouw, P. J. (2013). The therapeutic alliance: Exploring the concept of "safety" from a neuropsychotherapeutic perspective. *International Journal of Neuropsychotherapy, 1*, 21–29. doi:10.12744/ijnpt.2013.0021-0029

American Psychiatric Association. (2013). Depressive disorders. In *Diagnostic and statistical manual of mental disorders* (5th ed.). Washington, DC: American Psychiatric Publishing. doi:10.1176/appi.books.9780890425596.dsm04

Andrade, C., & Rao, N. S. K. (2010). How antidepressant drugs act: A primer on neuroplasticity as the eventual mediator of antidepressant efficacy. *Indian Journal of Psychiatry, 52*, 378–386. doi:10.4103/0019-5545.74318

Andrews, P. W., Bharwani, A., Lee, L. R., Fox, M., & Thomson, J. A., Jr. (2015). Is serotonin an upper or a downer? The evolution of the serotonergic system and its role in depression and the antidepressant response. *Neuroscience & Biobehavioral Reviews, 51*, 164–188. doi:10.1016/j.neubiorev.2015.01.018

Atkinson, R. C., & Shiffrin, R. M. (1968). Human memory: A proposed system and its control processes. In K. Spence & J. T. Spence (Eds.), *The psychology of learning and motivation* (Vol. 2, pp. 89–195). Oxford, United Kingdom: Academic Press. doi:10.1016/ S0079-7421(08)60422-3

Austin, M. A., Riniolo, T. C., & Porges, S. W. (2007). Borderline personality disorder and emotion regulation: Insights from the Polyvagal Theory. *Brain and Cognition, 65*, 69–76. 10.1016/j.bandc.2006.05.007

Baddeley, A., Eysenck, M. W., & Anderson, M. C. (2009). *Memory*. Oxford, United Kingdom: Psychology Press.

Badenoch, B. (2008). *Being a brain-wise therapist: A practical guide to interpersonal neurobiology*. New York, NY: W. W. Norton.

Baer, R. A., Smith, G. T., Hopkins, J., Krietemeyer, J., & Toney, L. (2006). Using self-report assessment methods to explore facets of mindfulness. *Assessment, 13*, 27–45. doi:10.1177/1073191105283504

Baratta, M. V., Kodandaramaiah, S. B., Monahan, P. E., Yao, J., Weber, M. D., Lin, P.-A., . . . Goosens, K. A. (2016). Stress enables reinforcement-elicited serotonergic consolidation of fear memory. *Biological Psychiatry, 79*, 814–822. doi:10.1016/j.biopsych.2015.06.025

Baylin, J. (2013, October). Behavioral epigenetics and attachment: The new science of trust and mistrust. *The Neuropsychotherapist, 3*, 68–79.

Becker, E. (1971). *The birth and death of meaning: An interdisciplinary perspective on the problem of man* (2nd ed.). Florence, MA: Free Press.

Benarroch, E. E. (2009). The locus ceruleus norepinephrine system: Functional organization and potential clinical significance. *Neurology, 73*, 1699–1704. doi:10.1212/WNL.0b013e3181c2937c

Bender, K. J., & Trussell, L. O. (2012). The physiology of the axon initial segment. *Annual Review of Neuroscience, 35*, 249–265. doi:10.1146/annurev-neuro-062111-150339

Bennett, B. T., Abee, C. R., & Henrickson, R. (Eds.). (1998). *Nonhuman primates in biomedical research: Diseases* (American College of Laboratory Animal Medicine; 1st ed.). Cambridge, MA: Academic Press.

Bewernick, B. H., Hurlemann, R., Matusch, A., Kayser,

S., Grubert, C., Hadrysiewicz, B., . . . Schlaepfer, T. E. (2010). Nucleus accumbens deep brain stimulation decreases ratings of depression and anxiety in treatment-resistant depression. *Biological Psychiatry, 67,* 110–116. doi:10.1016/j.biopsych.2009.09.013

Boden, J. M., Fergusson, D. M., & Horwood, L. J. (2008). Does adolescent self-esteem predict later life outcomes? A test of the causal role of self-esteem. *Development and Psychopathology, 20,* 319–339.

Bora, E., Fornito, A., Panetlis, C., & Yücel, M. (2011). Gray matter abnormalities in Major Depressive Disorder: A meta-analysis of voxel based morphometry studies. *Journal of Affective Disorders, 138,* 1–2, 9–18. doi:10.1016/j.jad.2011.03.049

Bowlby, J. (1973). *Attachment and loss* (Vol. 1): *Attachment.* New York, NY: Basic Books.

Bowlby, J. (1988). *A secure base: Parent–child attachment and healthy human development.* New York, NY: Basic Books.

Bravo, J. A., Forsythe, P., Chew, M. V., Escaravage, E., Savignac, H. M., Dinan, T. G., . . . Cryan, J. F. (2011). Ingestion of Lactobacillus strain regulates emotional behavior and central GABA receptor expression in a mouse via the vagus nerve. *Proceedings of the National Academy of Sciences, 108,* 16050–16055. doi:10.1073/pnas.1102999108

Bremner, J. D., Randall, P., Vermetten, E., Staib, L., Bronen, R. A., Mazure, C., . . . Charney, D. S. (1997). Magnetic resonance imaging-based measurement of hippocampal volume in posttraumatic stress disorder related to childhood physical and sexual abuse: A preliminary report. *Biological Psychiatry, 41,* 23–32.

Bromberg-Martin, E. S., & Hikosaka, O. (2011). Lateral habenula neurons signal errors in the prediction of reward information. *Nature Neuroscience, 14,* 1209–1216. doi:10.1038/nn.2902

Buckner, R. L., & Carroll, D. C. (2007). Self-projection and the brain. Trends in Cognitive Sciences, 11, 49–57. doi:10.1016/j.tics.2006.11.004

Buehlmann, E., Berger, G. E., Aston, J., Gschwandtner, U., Pflueger, M. O., Borgwardt, S. J., Radue, E. W., & Riecher-Rössler, A. (2010). Hippocampus abnormalities in at risk mental states for psychosis? A cross-sectional high resolution region of interest magnetic resonance imaging study. Journal of Psychiatric Research, 44, 447–453 doi:10.1016/j.jpsychires.2009.10.008

Busch, A. J., Barber, K. A. R., Overend, T. J., Peloso, P. M. J., & Schachter, C. L. (2007). Exercise for treating fibromyalgia syndrome. *Cochrane Database of Systematic Reviews,* Issue 4, Art. No. CD003786. doi:10.1002/14651858.CD003786.pub2

Buskila, D., & Cohen, H. (2007). Comorbidity of fibromyalgia and psychiatric disorders. *Current Pain and Headache Reports, 11,* 333–338. doi:10.1007/s11916-007-0214-4

Canli, T., Desmond, J. E., Zhao, Z., Glover, G., & Gabrieli, J. D. E. (1998). Hemispheric asymmetry for emotional stimuli detected with fMRI. *NeuroReport, 9,* 3233–3239.

Carr, L., Iacoboni, M., Dubeau, M. C., Maziotta, J. C., & Lenzi, L. G. (2003). Neural mechanisms of empathy in humans: A relay from neural systems for imitation to limbic areas. *Proceedings of the National Academy of Sciences, 100,* 5497–5502. doi:10.1073/pnas.0935845100

Caspi, A., Sugden, K., Moffitt, T. E., Taylor, A., Craig, I. W., Harrington, H., . . . Poulton, R. (2003). Influence of life stress on depression: Moderation by a polymorphism in the 5-HTT gene. *Science, 301*(5631), 386–389. doi:10.1126/science.1083968

Castrén, E., & Hen, R. (2013). Neuronal plasticity and antidepressant actions. *Trends in Neurosciences, 36,* 259–267. doi:10.1016/j.tins.2012.12.010

Castrén, E., Võikar, V., & Rantamäki, T. (2007). Role of neurotrophic factors in depression. *Current Opinion in Pharmacology, 7,* 18–21. doi:10.1016/j.coph.2006.08.009

Chakrabarty S, & Zoorob, R. (2007). Fibromyalgia. *American Family Physician, 76,* 247–254. Retrieved from http://www.aafp.org/afp/2007/0715/p247.html

Chang, Y.-S., Gratiot, M., Owen, J. P., Brandes-Aitken, A., Desai, S. S., Hill, S. S., . . . Mukherjee, P. (2016). White matter microstructure is associated with auditory and tactile processing in children with and without sensory processing disorder. *Frontiers in Neuroanatomy, 9:*169. doi:10.3389/fnana.2015.00169

Cheetham, S. C., Katona, C. L. E., & Horton, R. W. (1991). Post-mortem studies of neurotransmitter biochemistry in depression and suicide. In R. W. Horton & C. L. E. Katona (Eds.), *Biological aspects of affective disorders* (pp. 192–221). London, United Kingdom: Academic Press.

Cherney, K., & Holland, K. (2016, December 1). Everything you need to know about fibromyalgia [Web log post]. Retrieved from http://www.healthline.com/health/fibromyalgia

Clauw, D. J., Arnold, L. M., & McCarberg, B. H. (2011). The science of fibromyalgia. *Mayo Clinic Proceedings, 86*, 907–911. doi:10.4065/mcp.2011.0206

Clauw, D. J. (2014). Fibromyalgia: A clinical review. *JAMA, 311*, 1547–1555. doi:10.1001/jama.2014.3266

Comb, M., & Goodman, H. M. (1990). CpG methylation inhibits proenkephalin gene expression and binding of the transcription factor AP-2. *Nucleic Acids Research, 18*, 3975–3982.

Cozolino, L. (2013). The social neuroscience of education: Optimizing attachment and learning in the classroom. New York, NY: W. W. Norton.

Cozolino, L. (2014). *The neuroscience of human relationships: Attachment and the developing social brain* (2nd ed.). New York, NY: W. W. Norton.

Craig, J. B., & Lindsay, N. J. (2001). Quantifying "gut feeling" in the opportunity recognition process. In W. Bygrave, E. Autio, C. G. Brush, P. Davidsson, P. G. Green, P. D. Reynolds, & H. J. Sapienza (Eds.), *Frontiers of entrepreneurship research: Proceedings of the twenty-first annual Entrepreneurship Research Conference* (pp. 124–137). Wellesley, MA: Babson College.

Craik, F. I. M., & Lockhart, R. S. (1972). Levels of processing: A framework for memory research. *Journal of Verbal Learning and Verbal Behavior, 11*, 671–684.

Cryan, J. F., & O'Mahony, S. M. (2011). The microbiome–gut–brain axis: From bowel to behavior. *Neurogastroenterology & Motility, 23*, 187–192.

Csikszentmihalyi, M. (1991). *Flow: The psychology of optimal experience.* New York, NY: Harper Perennial.

Dahlitz, M. J., & Rossouw, P. J. (2014). The consistency-theoretical model of mental functioning: Towards a refined perspective. In P. J. Rossouw (Ed.), *Neuropsychotherapy: Theoretical underpinnings and clinical applications.* Brisbane, Australia: Mediros.

Dane, E., & Pratt, M. G. (2007). Exploring intuition and its role in managerial decision making. *Academy of Management Review, 32*, 33–54. doi:10.5465/AMR.2007.23463682

Danese, A., & Baldwin, J. R. (2017). Hidden wounds? Inflammatory links between childhood trauma and psychopathology. *Annual Review of Psychology, 68*, 517–544. doi:10.1146/annurev-psych-010416-044208

Dapretto, M., Davies, M. S., Pfeifer, J. H., Scott, A. A., Sigman, M., Bookheimer, S. Y., & Iacoboni, M. (2006). Understanding emotions in others: Mirror neuron dysfunction in children with autism spectrum disorders. *Nature Neuroscience, 9*, 28–30.

Davidson, R. J. (1992). Emotion and affective style: Hemispheric substrates. *Psychological Science, 3*, 39–43.

Davidson, R. J. (2000). Affective style, psychopathology, and resilience: Brain mechanisms and plasticity. *American Psychologist, 55*, 1196–1214.

Davidson, R. J., & Henriques, J. B. (2000). Regional brain function in sadness and depression. In J. C. Borod (Ed.), *The neuropsychology of emotion* (pp. 269–297). New York, NY: Oxford University Press.

Davidson, R. J., Pizzagalli, D., Nitschke, J. B., & Putnam, K. (2002). Depression: Perspectives from affective neuroscience. *Annual Review of Psychology, 53*, 545–574.

Desbonnet, L., Garrett, L., Clarke, G., Bienenstock, J., & Dinan, T. G. (2008). The probiotic Bifidobacteria infantis: An assessment of potential antidepressant properties in the rat. *Journal of Psychiatric Research, 43*, 164–174.

DeWall, C. N., MacDonald, G., Webster, G. D., Masten, C. L., Baumeister, R. F., Powell, C., . . . Eisenberger, N. I. (2010). Acetaminophen reduces social pain: Behavioral and neural evidence. *Psychological Science, 21*, 931–937. doi:10.1177/0956797610374741

Diamond, A. (2013). Executive functions. *Annual Review of Psychology, 64*, 135–168. doi:10.1146/annurev-psych-113011-143750

DiGangi, J. A., Tadayyon, A., Fitzgerald, D. A., Rabinak, C. A., Kennedy, A., Klumpp, H., . . . Phan, K. L. (2016). Reduced default mode network connectivity following combat trauma. *Neuroscience Letters, 615*, 37–43. doi:10.1016/j.neulet.2016.01.010

Dinan, T. G., & Cryan, J. F. (2013). Melancholic microbes: A link between gut microbiota and depression? *Neurogastroenterology & Motility, 25*, 713–719. doi:10.1111/nmo.12198

Drachman, D. A. (2005). Do we have brain to spare? *Neurology, 64*, 2004–2005. doi:10.1212/01.WNL.0000166914.38327.BB

Duman, R. S., & Aghajanian, G. K. (2012). Synaptic dysfunction in depression: Potential therapeutic targets. *Science, 338*(6103), 68–72. doi:10.1126/science.1222939

Duman, R. S., & Voleti, B. (2012). Signaling pathways underlying the pathophysiology and treatment of depression: Novel mechanisms for rapid-acting agents. *Trends in Neurosciences, 35*, 47–56.

doi:10.1016/j.tins.2011.11.004

Ecker, B. (2015). Memory reconsolidation understood and misunderstood. *International Journal of Neuropsychotherapy, 3*, 2–46. doi:10.12744/ijnpt.2015.0002-0046

Ecker, B., Ticic, R., & Hulley, L. (2012). *Unlocking the emotional brain: Eliminating symptoms at their roots using memory reconsolidation.* New York, NY: Routledge.

Eisch, A. J., & Petrik, D. (2012). Depression and hippocampal neurogenesis: A road to remission? *Science, 338*(6103), 72–75. doi:10.1126/science.1222941

Eisenberger, N. I. (2012). The neural bases of social pain: Evidence for shared representations with physical pain. *Psychosomatic Medicine, 74*, 126–135. doi:10.1097/PSY.0b013e3182464dd1

Eisenberger, N. I., Lieberman, M. D., & Williams, K. D. (2003). Does rejection hurt? An fMRI study of social exclusion. *Science, 302*(5643), 290–292. doi:10.1126/science.1089134

Elliot, A. J. (2006). The hierarchical model of approach-avoidance motivation. *Motivation and Emotion, 30*, 111–116.

Elliot, A. J. (2008). *Handbook of approach and avoidance motivation.* New York, NY: Psychology Press.

Epstein, S. (1973). The self-concept revisited, or a theory of a theory. *American Psychologist, 28*, 404–416

Epstein, S. (1980). The self-concept: A review and the proposal of an integrated theory of personality. In E. Staub (Ed.), *Personality: Basic issues and current research* (pp. 82–132). Englewood Cliffs, NJ: Prentice Hall.

Epstein, S. (1990). Cognitive-experiential self-theory. In L. A. Pervin (Ed.), *Handbook of personality: Theory and research* (pp. 165–192). New York, NY: Guilford Press.

Epstein, S. (1991). Cognitive–experiential self-theory: An integrative theory of personality. In R. Curtis (Ed.), *The relational self: Convergences in psychoanalysis and social psychology* (pp. 111–137). New York, NY: Guilford Press.

Epstein, S. (1993). Implications of cognitive–experiential self-theory for personality and developmental psychology. In D. Funder, R. Parke, C. Tomlinson-Keasey, & K. Widamen (Eds.), *Studying lives through time: Personality and development* (pp. 399–438). Washington, DC: American Psychological Association.

Epstein, S. (1994). Integration of the cognitive and the psychodynamic unconscious. *American Psychologist, 49*, 709–724.

Epstein, S. (1998). Cognitive–experiential self-theory. In D. F. Barone, M. Hersen, & V. B. Van Hasselt (Eds.), *Advanced personality* (pp. 212–238). New York, NY: Springer.

Evrensel, A., & Ceylan, M. E. (2015). The gut–brain axis: The missing link in depression. *Clinical Psychopharmacology and Neuroscience, 13*, 239–244. doi:10.9758/cpn.2015.13.3.239

Fales, C. L., Barch, D. M., Rundle, M. M., Mintun, M. A., Mathews, J., Snyder, A. Z., & Sheline, Y. I. (2009). Antidepressant treatment normalizes hypoactivity in dorsolateral prefrontal cortex during emotional interference processing in major depression. *Journal of Affective Disorders, 112*, 206–211. doi:10.1016/j.jad.2008.04.027

Fang, J., Rong, P., Hong, Y., Fan, Y., Liu, J., Wang, H., . . . Kong, J. (2016). Transcutaneous vagus nerve stimulation modulates default mode network in major depressive disorder. *Biological Psychiatry, 79*, 266–273. doi:10.1016/j.biopsych.2015.03.025

Flückiger, C., & Grosse Holtforth, M. (2008). Focusing the therapist's attention on the patient's strengths: A preliminary study to foster a mechanism of change in outpatient psychotherapy. *Journal of Clinical Psychology, 64*, 876–890.

Flückiger, C., Caspar, F., Grosse Holtforth, M., & Willutzki, U. (2009). Working with patients' strengths: A microprocess approach. *Psychotherapy Research, 19*, 213–223.

Flückiger, C., Wüsten, G., Zinbarg, R. E., & Wampold, B. E. (2009). *Resource activation: Using clients' own strengths in psychotherapy and counseling.* Cambridge, MA: Hogrefe & Huber.

Fox, M. D., Snyder, A. Z., Vincent, J. L., Corbetta, M., van Essen, D. C., & Raichle, M. E. (2005). The human brain is intrinsically organised into dynamic, anticorrelated functional networks. *Proceedings of the National Academy of Sciences, 102*, 9673–9678. doi:10.1073/pnas.0504136102

Freud, S. (1959). Beyond the pleasure principle. New York, NY: W. W. Norton. (Original work published 1920)

Frodl, T., Möller, H.-J., & Meisenzahl, E. (2008). Neuroimaging genetics: New perspectives in research on major depression? *Acta Psychiatrica Scandinavica, 118*, 363–372. doi:10.1111/j.1600-0447.2008.01225.x

Fusar-Poli, P., Perez, J., Broome, M., Borgwardt, S., Placentino, A., Caverzasi, E., . . . McGuire, P. (2007). Neurofunctional correlates of vulnerability to psychosis: A systematic review and meta-analysis. *Neuroscience & Biobehavioral Reviews, 31*, 465–484. doi:10.1016/j.neubiorev.2006.11.006

Gallese, V., Fadiga, L., Fogassi, L., & Rizzolati, G. (1996). Action recognition in the premotor cortex. *Brain, 119*, 593–609.

Gassmann, D., & Grawe, K. (2006). General change mechanisms: The relation between problem activation and resource activation in successful and unsuccessful therapeutic interactions. *Clinical Psychology and Psychotherapy, 13*, 1–11. doi:10.1002/cpp.442

Gatt, J. M., Williams, L. M., Schofield, P. R., Dobson-Stone, C., Paul, R. H., Grieve, S. M., . . . Nemeroff, C. B. (2010). Impact of the HTR3A gene with early life trauma on emotional brain networks and depressed mood. *Depression and Anxiety, 27*, 752–759. doi:10.1002/da.20726

Geuze, E., Vermetten, E., & Bremner, J. D. (2005). MR-based in vivo hippocampal volumetrics: 2. Findings in neuropsychiatric disorders. *Molecular Psychiatry, 10*, 160–184. doi:10.1038/sj.mp.4001579

Gill, S. R., Pop, M., Deboy, R. T., Eckburg, P. B., Turnbaugh, P. J., Samuel, B. S., . . . Nelson, K. E. (2006). Metagenomic analysis of the human distal gut microbiome. *Science, 312*(5778), 1355–1359. doi:10.1126/science.1124234

Gjerris, A. (1988). Baseline studies on transmitter substances in cerebrospinal fluid in depression. *Acta Psychiatrica Scandinavica, 78*, 1–35. doi:10.1111/j.1600-0447.1988.tb10571.x

Glass, J. M. (2006). Cognitive dysfunction in fibromyalgia and chronic fatigue syndrome: New trends and future directions. *Current Rheumatology Reports, 8*, 425–429. doi:10.1007/s11926-006-0036-0

Goff, B., Gee, D. G., Telzer, E. H., Humphreys, K. L., Gabard-Durnam, L., Flannery, J., & Tottenham, N. (2013). Reduced nucleus accumbens reactivity and adolescent depression following early-life stress. *Neuroscience, 249*, 129–138.

Gowans, S. E., & deHueck, A. (2004). Effectiveness of exercise in management of fibromyalgia. *Current Opinion in Rheumatology, 16*, 138–142. doi:10.1097/00002281-200403000-00012

Grawe, K. (2004). *Psychological therapy.* Toronto, Canada: Hogrefe & Huber.

Grawe, K. (2007). *Neuropsychotherapy: How the neurosciences inform effective psychotherapy.* New York, NY: Psychology Press.

Grenham, S., Clarke, G., Cryan, J. F., & Dinan, T. G. (2011). Brain–gut–microbe communication in health and disease. *Frontiers in Physiology, 2*, 94. doi:10.3389/fphys.2011.00094

Grieve, S. M., Korgaonkar, M. S., Koslow, S. H., Gordon, E., & Williams, L. M. (2013). Widespread reductions in gray matter volume in depression. *NeuroImage: Clinical, 3*, 332–339. doi:10.1016/j.nicl.2013.08.016

Groves, J. O. (2007). Is it time to reassess the BDNF hypothesis of depression? *Molecular Psychiatry, 12*, 1079–1088. doi:10.1038/sj.mp.4002075

Grunstein, M. (1997). Histone acetylation in chromatin structure and transcription. *Nature, 389*, 349–352. doi:10.1038/38664

Guillemin, G. J. (2012). Quinolinic acid, the inescapable neurotoxin. *The FEBS Journal, 279*, 1356–1365. doi:10.1111/j.1742-4658.2012.08485.x

Haapakoski, R., Mathieu, J., Ebmeier, K. P., Alenius, H., & Kivimäki, M. (2015). Cumulative meta-analysis of interleukins 6 and 1β, tumour necrosis factor α and C-reactive protein in patients with major depressive disorder. *Brain, Behavior, and Immunity, 49*, 206–215. doi:10.1016/j.bbi.2015.06.001

Habib, M. (2004). Athymhormia and disorders of motivation in basal ganglia disease. *The Journal of Neuropsychiatry and Clinical Neurosciences, 16*, 509–524. doi:10.1176/jnp.16.4.509

Hajcak, G., Moser, J. S., Holroyd, C. B., & Simons R. F. (2006). The feedback-related negativity reflects the binary evaluation of good versus bad outcomes. *Biological Psychology, 71*, 148–154. doi:10.1016/j.biopsycho.2005.04.001

Hamilton, J. P., Farmer, M., Fogelman, P., & Gotlib, I. H. (2015). Depressive rumination, the default-mode network, and the dark matter of clinical neuroscience. *Biological Psychiatry, 78*, 224–230. doi:10.1016/j.biopsych.2015.02.020

Hamilton, J. P., Siemer, M., & Gotlib, I. H. (2008). Amygdala volume in Major Depressive Disorder: A meta-analysis of magnetic resonance imaging studies. *Molecular Psychiatry, 13*, 993–1000. doi:10.1038/mp.2008.57

Hariri, A. R., Goldberg, T. E., Mattay, V. S., Kolachana, B. S., Callicott, J. H., Egan, M. F., & Weinberger, D. R. (2003). Brain-derived neurotrophic factor Val-66Met polymorphism affects human memory-related hippocampal activity and predicts memory performance. *Journal of Neuroscience, 23*, 6690–6694.

Häuser, W., Bernardy, K., Uçeyler, N., & Sommer, C. (2009). Treatment of fibromyalgia syndrome with antidepressants: A meta-analysis. *JAMA, 301*, 198–209. doi:10.1001/jama.2008.944

Hawkins, J., & Blakeslee, S. (2004). *On intelligence: How a new understanding of the brain will lead to the creation of truly intelligent machines.* New York, NY: Times Books.

Hawkins, R. A. (2013). Fibromyalgia: A clinical update. *The Journal of the American Osteopathic Association, 113*, 680–689. doi:10.7556/jaoa.2013.034

Healy, D., & Leonard, B. E. (1987). Monoamine transport in depression: Kinetics and dynamics. *Journal of Affective Disorders, 12*, 91–103.

Henriques, J. B., & Davidson, R. J. (2000). Decreased responsiveness to reward in depression. *Cognition and Emotion, 14*, 711–724. doi:10.1080/02699930050117684

Heshmati, M., & Russo, S. J. (2015). Anhedonia and the brain reward circuitry in depression. *Current Behavioral Neuroscience Reports, 2*, 146–153. doi:10.1007/s40473-015-0044-3

Higuera, V. (2016, August 17). Fibromyalgia: Real or imagined? [Web log post]. Retrieved from http://www.healthline.com/health/fibromyalgia-real-or-imagined

Hill, R. (2013, April). Malleable genetics. *The Neuropsychotherapist, 1*, 102–103.

Ho, T. C., Connolly, C. G., Blom, E. H., LeWinn, K. Z., Strigo, I. A., Paulus, M. P., . . . Yang, T. T. (2015). Emotion-dependent functional connectivity of the default mode network in adolescent depression. *Biological Psychiatry, 78*, 635–646. doi:10.1016/j.biopsych.2014.09.002

Holtzheimer, P. E., Kelley, M. E., Gross, R. E., Filkowski, M. M., Garlow, S. J., Barrocas, A., . . . Mayberg, H. S. (2012). Subcallosal cingulate deep brain stimulation for treatment-resistant unipolar and bipolar depression. *Archives of General Psychiatry, 69*, 150–158. doi:10.1001/archgenpsychiatry.2011.1456

Hsu, D. T., Sanford, B. J., Meyers, K. K., Love, T. M., Hazlett, K. E., Wang, H., . . . Zubieta, J.-K. (2013). Response of the μ-opioid system to social rejection and acceptance. *Molecular Psychiatry, 18*, 1211–1217. doi:10.1038/mp.2013.96

Iacoboni, M., Koski, L. M., Brass, M., Bekkering, H., Woods, R. P., Dubeau, M., . . . Rizzolati, G. (2001). Reafferent copies of imitated actions in the right superior temporal cortex. *Proceedings of the National Academy of Sciences, 98*, 13995–13999. doi:10.1073/pnas.241474598

Iannetti, G. D., Salomons, T. V., Moayedi, M., Mouraux, A., & Davis, K. D. (2013). Beyond metaphor: Contrasting mechanisms of social and physical pain. *Trends in Cognitive Sciences, 17*, 371–378. doi:10.1016/j.tics.2013.06.002

Kabat-Zinn, J. (1994). *Wherever you go there you are: Mindfulness meditation in everyday life* (10th anniversary ed.). New York, NY: Hyperion.

Kabat-Zinn, J. (2013). *Full catastrophe living: Using the wisdom of your body and mind to face stress, pain, and illness* (Rev. ed.). New York, NY: Bantam Books.

Kaminsky, Z. A., Tang, T., Wang, S., Ptak, C., Oh, G. H., Wong, A. H., . . . Petronis, A. (2009). DNA methylation profiles in monozygotic and dizygotic twins. *Nature Genetics, 41*, 240–245. doi:10.1038/ng.286

Kandel, E. R. (2006). *In search of memory: The emergence of a new science of mind.* New York, NY: W. W. Norton.

Kandel, E. R. (2013, December 10). We are what we remember: Memory and the biological basis of individuality [Video file]. Retrieved from https://youtu.be/skyvzMxtLu8

Kandel, E. R., Schwartz, J. H., Jessell, T. M., Siegelbaum, S. A., & Hudspeth, A. J. (Eds.). (2012). *Principles of neural science* (5th ed.). New York, NY: McGraw-Hill.

Karg, K., Burmeister, M., Shedden, K., & Sen, S. (2011). The serotonin transporter promoter variant (5-HT-TLPR), stress, and depression meta-analysis revisited: Evidence of genetic moderation. *Archives of General Psychiatry, 68*, 444–454. doi:10.1001/archgenpsychiatry.2010.189

Kauffman, A., & Meaney, M. J. (2007). Neurodevelopmental sequelae of postnatal maternal care in rodents: Clinical and research implications of molecular insights. *Journal of Child Psychology and Psychiatry, 48*, 224–244.

Keleman, S. (2013, January 6). Slow attending: The art of forming intimacy [Web log post]. Retrieved from http://www.neuropsychotherapist.com/slow-attending-article

Kempton, M. J., Salvador, Z., Munafò, M. R., Geddes, J. R., Simmons, A., Frangou, S., & Williams, S. C. R. (2011). Structural neuroimaging studies in major depressive disorder: Meta-analysis and comparison with bipolar disorder. *Archives of General Psychiatry, 68,* 675–690. doi:10.1001/archgenpsychiatry.2011.60

Keysers, C. (2011). *The empathic brain: How the discovery of mirror neurons changes our understanding of human nature* [Kindle reader version]. Retrieved from https://www.amazon.com/Empathic-Brain-Christian-Keysers-ebook/dp/B0054S7DOO

Kiliaan, A. J., Saunders, P. R., Bijlsma, P. B., Berin, M. C., Taminiau, J. A., Groot, J. A., & Perdue, M. H. (1998). Stress stimulates transepithelial macromolecular uptake in rat jejunum. *American Journal of Physiology, 275,* G1037–G1044.

Kitamura, T., Ogawa, S. K., Roy, D. S., Okuyama, T., Morrissey, M. D., Smith, L. M., . . . Tonegawa, S. (2017). Engrams and circuits crucial for systems consolidation of a memory. *Science, 356*(6333), 73–78. doi:10.1126/science.aam6808

Konishi, M., McLaren, D. G., Engen, H., & Smallwood, J. (2015). Shaped by the past: The default mode network supports cognition that is independent of immediate perceptual input. *PLoS One, 10*: e0132209. doi:10.1371/journal.pone.0132209

Lacey, B. C., & Lacey J. I. (1974). Studies of heart rate and other bodily processes in sensorimotor behavior. In P. A. Obrist, A. H. Black, J. Brener, & L. V. DiCara (Eds.), *Cardiovascular psychophysiology* (pp. 538–564). Chicago, IL: Aldine.

Lambert, K. G., & Kinsley, C. H. (2004). *Clinical neuroscience: The neurobiological foundations of mental health.* New York, NY: Worth.

Lambert, K. G., & Kinsley, C. H. (2010). *Clinical neuroscience: Psychopathology and the brain* (2nd ed.). Melbourne, Australia: Oxford University Press.

Langer, E. J., & Rodin, J. (1976). The effects of choice and enhanced personal responsibility for the aged: A field experiment in an institutional setting. *Journal of Personality and Social Psychology, 34,* 191–198.

Lavater, J. C. (1832). *The pocket Lavater, or, The science of physiognomy: to which is added, An inquiry into the analogy existing between brute and human physiognomy, from the Italian of Porta.* Hartford: Andrus & Judd. Digitally rendered version retrieved from https://archive.org/details/56910710R.nlm.nih.gov

Lawson, R. P., Nord, C. L., Seymour, B., Thomas, D. L., Dayan, P., Pilling, S., & Roiser, J. P. (2017). Disrupted habenula function in major depression. *Molecular Psychiatry, 22,* 202–208. doi:10.1038/mp.2016.81

Leavitt, F., Katz, R. S., Mills, M., & Heard, A. R. (2002). Cognitive and dissociative manifestations in fibromyalgia. *Journal of Clinical Rheumatology, 8,* 77–84. doi:10.1097/00124743-200204000-00003

Leotti, L. A., & Delgado, M. (2011). The inherent reward of choice. *Psychological Science, 22,* 1310–1318. doi:10.1177/0956797611417005

Leotti, L. A., Iyengar, S. S., & Ochsner, K., N. (2010). Born to choose: The origins and value of the need for control. *Trends in Cognitive Sciences, 14,* 457–463. doi:10.1016/j.tics.2010.08.001

Lesch, K.-P., Bengel, D., Heils, A., Sabol, S. Z., Greenberg, B. D., Petri, S., . . . Murphy, D. L. (1996). Association of anxiety-related traits with a polymorphism in the serotonin transporter gene regulatory region. *Science, 274*(5292), 1527–1531. doi:10.1126/science.274.5292.1527

Levenson, J. M., & Sweatt, J. D. (2005). Epigenetic mechanisms in memory formation. *Nature Reviews Neuroscience, 6,* 108–118. doi:10.1038/nrn1604

Lewis, R., Asplin, K. E., Bruce, G., Dart, C., Mobasheri, A., & Barrett-Jolley, R. (2011). The role of the membrane potential in chondrocyte volume regulation. *Journal of Cellular Physiology, 226,* 2979–2986. doi:10.1002/jcp.22646

Ley, R. E., Peterson, D. A., & Gordon, J. I. (2006). Ecological and evolutionary forces shaping microbial diversity in the human intestine. *Cell, 124,* 837–848. doi:10.1016/j.cell.2006.02.017

Lieberman, M. D. (2013). *Social: Why our brains are wired to connect.* New York, NY: Crown.

Lindauer, R. J., Vlieger, E. J., Jalink, M., Olff, M., Carlier, I. V., Majoie, C. B., . . . Gersons, B. P. (2005). Effects of psychotherapy on hippocampal volume in out-patients with post-traumatic stress disorder: An MRI investigation. *Psychological Medicine, 10,* 1421–1431. doi:10.1017/S0033291705005246

Linden, D. E. J. (2006). How psychotherapy changes the brain: The contribution of functional neuroimaging. *Molecular Psychiatry, 11,* 528–538. doi:10.1038/sj.mp.4001816

Lozano, A. M., Giacobbe, P., Hamani, C., Rizvi, S. J., Kennedy, S. H., Kolivakis, T. T., . . . Mayberg, H. S. (2012). A multicenter pilot study of subcallosal cingulate area deep brain stimulation for treatment-resistant depression. *Journal of Neurosurgery, 116,* 315–322. doi:10.3171/2011.10.JNS102122

Lozano, A. M., Mayberg, H. S., Giacobbe, P., Hamani, C., Craddock, R. C., & Kennedy, S. H. (2008). Subcallosal cingulate gyrus deep brain stimulation for treatment-resistant depression. *Biological Psychiatry, 64*, 461–467. doi:10.1016/j.biopsych.2008.05.034

Luby, J. L., Belden, A. C., Jackson. J. J., Lessov-Schlaggar, C. N., Harms, M. P., Tillman, R., . . . Barch, D. M. (2016). Early childhood depression and alterations in the trajectory of gray matter maturation in middle childhood and early adolescence. *JAMA Psychiatry, 73*, 31–38. doi:10.1001/jamapsychiatry.2015.2356

Lundqvist, L., & Dimberg, U. (1995). Facial expressions are contagious. *Journal of Psycophysiology, 9*, 203–211.

Lupien, S. J., McEwen, B. S., Gunnar, M. R., & Heim, C. (2009). Effects of stress throughout the lifespan on the brain, behaviour and cognition. *Nature Reviews Neuroscience, 10*, 434–445. doi:10.1038/nrn2639

MacLean, P. D. (1990). *The triune brain in evolution: Role in paleocerebral functions.* New York, NY: Plenum Press.

Maguire, E. A. (2008, November 25). Mapping memory: The brains behind remembering [Video file]. Retrieved from https://youtu.be/JW23BPngkQ8

Main, M., & Solomon, J. (1986). Discovery of an insecure-disorganized/disoriented attachment pattern. In T. B. Brazelton & M. Yogaman (Eds.), *Affective development in infancy* (pp. 95–124). Norwood, NJ: Ablex.

Malenka, R. C., Nestler, E. J., & Hyman, S.E. (2009). Widely projecting systems: Monoamines, acetylcholine, and orexin. In A. Sydor & R. Y. Brown (Eds.), *Molecular neuropharmacology: A foundation for clinical neuroscience* (2nd ed., pp. 145–180). New York, NY: McGraw-Hill.

Maletic, V., & Raison, C. L. (2009). Neurobiology of depression, fibromyalgia and neuropathic pain [Special issue]. *Frontiers in Bioscience, 14*, 5291–5338. doi:10.2741/3598

Matsumoto, M., & Hikosaka, O. (2007). Lateral habenula as a source of negative reward signals in dopamine neurons. *Nature, 447*(7148), 1111–1115. doi:10.1038/nature05860

Matthews, P. R., & Harrison, P. J. (2012). A morphometric, immunohistochemical, and in situ hybridization study of the dorsal raphe nucleus in major depression, bipolar disorder, schizophrenia, and suicide. *Journal of Affective Disorders, 137*, 125–134. doi:10.1016/j.jad.2011.10.043

Mawe, G. M., & Hoffman, J. M. (2013). Serotonin signalling in the gut: Functions, dysfunctions and therapeutic targets. *Nature Reviews Gastroenterology & Hepatology, 10*, 473–486. doi:10.1038/nrgastro.2013.105

Mayer, E. A. (2011). Gut feelings: The emerging biology of gut–brain communication. *Nature Reviews Neuroscience, 12*, 453–466. doi:10.1038/nrn3071

Mayer, E. A., Knight, R., Mazmanian, S. K., Cryan, J. F., & Tillisch, K. (2014). Gut microbes and the brain: Paradigm shift in neuroscience. *Journal of Neuroscience, 34*, 15490–15496. doi:10.1523/JNEUROSCI.3299-14.2014

McCandless, P. (1992). Mesmerism and phrenology in antebellum Charleston: "Enough of the marvellous". *Journal of Southern History, 58*, 199–230.

McCraty, R. (2015a). Heart–brain neurodynamics: The making of emotions. In M. Dahlitz & G. Hall (Eds.), *An issue of the heart* [Special issue of *The Neuropsychotherapist*] (pp. 76–110). Brisbane, Australia: Dahlitz Media.

McCraty, R. (2015b). *Science of the heart: Exploring the role of the heart in human performance* (Vol. 2). Boulder Creek, CA: HeartMath Institute. Retrieved from https://www.heartmath.org/research/science-of-the-heart/

McDougall, W. (1936). *An introduction to social psychology* (Rev. ed.). London, United Kingdom: Methuen.

McGilchrist, I. (2009). *The master and his emissary: The divided brain and the making of the Western world.* New Haven, CT: Yale University Press.

McKim, D. B., Patterson, J. M., Wohleb, E. S., Jarrett, B. L., Reader, B. F., Godbout, J. P., & Sheridan, J. F. (2016). Sympathetic release of splenic monocytes promotes recurring anxiety following repeated social defeat. *Biological Psychiatry, 79*, 803–813. doi:10.1016/j.biopsych.2015.07.010

Meltzoff, A. N., Kuhl, P. K., Movellan, J., & Sejnowski, T. J. (2009). Foundations for a new science of learning. *Science, 325*(5938), 284–288. doi:10.1126/science.1175626

Meyer, P. W., Müller, L. E., Zastrow, A., Schmidinger, I., Bohus, M., Herpertz, S. C., & Bertsch, K. (2016). Heart rate variability in patients with post-traumatic stress disorder or borderline personality disorder: Relationship to early life maltreatment. *Journal of Neural Transmission,123*, 1107–1118. doi:10.1007/s00702-016-1584-8

Milham, M (2003). Practice-related effects demonstrate complementary roles of anterior cingulate and prefrontal cortices in attentional control. *NeuroImage, 18*, 483–493. doi:10.1016/s1053-8119(02)00050-2.

Miller, G. A. (1956). The magical number seven, plus or minus two: Some limits on our capacity for processing information. *Psychological Review, 63*, 81–97.

Modell, J. G., Mountz, J. M., Curtis, G. C., & Greden, J. F. (1989). Neurophysiologic dysfunction in basal ganglia/limbic striatal and thalamocortical circuits as a pathogenetic mechanism of obsessive–compulsive disorder. *Journal of Neuropsychiatry & Clinical Neuroscience, 1*, 27–36. doi:10.1176/jnp.1.1.27

Moss, R. A. (2006). Of bits and logic: Cortical columns in learning and memory. *The Journal of Mind and Behavior, 27*, 215–246.

Moss, R. A. (2007). Negative emotional memories in clinical practice: Theoretical considerations. *Journal of Psychotherapy Integration, 17*, 209–224.

Moss, R. A. (2014). Brain-based views on psychotherapy integration: Clinical biopsychology. *New Therapist, 89*, 6–15.

Moss, R. A. (2016, February). The hippocampus and memory: The binding of parallel cortical circuits. *The Neuropsychotherapist, 4*(2), 16–19.

Moss, R. A., & Mahan, M. C. (2014). Emotional restructuring: Clinical biopsychological perspective on brain involvement. *The Neuropsychotherapist, 5*, 54–65. doi:10.12744/tnpt(5)054-065

Moss, R. A., & Moss, J. (2014a). The role of cortical columns in explaining gamma-band synchronization and NMDA receptors in cognitive functions. *AIMS Neuroscience, 1*, 65–88. doi:10.3934/Neuroscience2014.1.65

Moss, R. A., & Moss, J. (2014b). Commentary on the Pinotsis and Friston neural fields DCM and the Cadonic and Albensi oscillations and NMDA receptors articles. *AIMS Neuroscience, 1*, 158–162. doi:10.3934/Neuroscience.2014.2.158

Nader, K., & Hardt, O. (2009). A single standard for memory: The case for reconsolidation. *Nature Reviews Neuroscience, 10*, 224–234. doi:10.1038/nrn2590

Naranjo, C. A., Tremblay, L. K., & Busto, U. E. (2001). The role of the brain reward system in depression. *Progress in Neuro-Psychopharmacology & Biological Psychiatry, 25*, 781–823.

Nemeroff, C. B. (1998, June). The neurobiology of depression. *Scientific American, 278*(6), 42–49. doi:10.1038/scientificamerican0698-42

Ngian, G.-S., Guymer, E. K., & Littlejohn, G. O. (2011). The use of opioids in fibromyalgia. *International Journal of Rheumatic Diseases, 14*, 6–11.

doi:10.1111/j.1756-185X.2010.01567.x

Nieuwenhuis, S., Slagter, H. A., Von Geusau, N. J. A., Heslenfeld, D. J., & Holroyd, C. B. (2005), Knowing good from bad: Differential activation of human cortical areas by positive and negative outcomes. *European Journal of Neuroscience, 21*, 3161–3168. doi:10.1111/j.1460-9568.2005.04152.x

O'Keefe, J., & Dostrovsky, J. (1971). The hippocampus as a spatial map: Preliminary evidence from unit activity in the freely moving rat. *Brain Research, 34*, 171–175. doi:10.1016/0006-8993(71)90358-1

Okifuji, A., & Hare, B. D. (2013). Management of fibromyalgia syndrome: Review of evidence. *Pain and Therapy, 2*, 87–104. doi:10.1007/s40122-013-0016-9

Orth, U., Robins, R. W., & Roberts, B. W. (2008). Low self-esteem prospectively predicts depression in adolescence and young adulthood. *Journal of Personality and Social Psychology, 95*, 695–708.

Palazidou, E. (2012). The neurobiology of depression. *British Medical Bulletin, 101*, 127–145. doi:10.1093/bmb/lds004

Panksepp, J., & Biven, L. (2012). *The archaeology of mind: Neuroevolutionary origins of human emotions.* New York, NY: W. W. Norton.

Paradiso, S., Johnson, D. L., Andreasen, N. C., O'Leary, D. S., Watkins, G. L., Ponto, L. L. B., & Hichwa, R. D. (1999). Cerebral blood flow changes associated with attribution of emotional valence to pleasant, unpleasant, and neural visual stimuli in a PET study of normal subjects. *American Journal of Psychiatry, 156*, 1618–1629. doi:10.1176/ajp.156.10.1618

Park, L. E., & Crocker, J. (2013). Pursuing self-esteem: Implications for self-regulation and relationships. In V. Zeigler-Hill (Ed.), *Self-esteem* (pp. 43–59). Florence, KY: Psychology Press.

Partanen, E., Kujala, T., Näätänen, R., Liitola, A., Sambeth, A., & Huotilainen, M. (2013). Learning-induced neural plasticity of speech processing before birth. *Proceedings of the National Academy of Sciences, 110*, 15145–15150. doi:10.1073/pnas.1302159110

Peckham, H. (2013). Epigenetics: The dogma-defying discovery that genes learn from experience. *International Journal of Neuropsychotherapy, 1*, 9–20. doi:10.12744/ijnpt.2013.0009-0020

Peckham, H. (2015). The unexpected interdependence of heart and mind. In M. Dahlitz & G. Hall (Eds.), *An issue of the heart* [Special issue of *The Neuropsychotherapist*] (pp. 111–118). Brisbane, Australia: Dahlitz Media.

Perkins, T., Stokes, M., McGillivray, J., & Bittar, R. (2010). Mirror neuron dysfunction in autism spectrum disorders. *Journal of Clinical Neuroscience, 17*, 1239–1243. doi:10.1016/j.jocn.2010.01.026

Piccinni, A., Del Debbio, A., Medda, P., Bianchi, C., Roncaglia, I., Veltri, A., . . . Dell'Osso, L. (2009). Plasma brain-derived neurotrophic factor in treatment-resistant depressed patients receiving electroconvulsive therapy. *European Neuropsychopharmacology, 19*, 349–355. doi:10.1016/j.euroneuro.2009.01.002

Pinel, P. J., & Barnes, S. J. (2012). *Introduction to biopsychology* (9th ed.). Essex, United Kingdom: Pearson Education.

Popoli, M., Yan, Z., McEwen, B. S., & Sanacora, G. (2012). The stressed synapse: The impact of stress and glucocorticoids on glutamate transmission. *Nature Reviews Neuroscience, 13*, 22–37. doi:10.1038/nrn3138

Porges, S. (2011). *The polyvagal theory: Neurophysiological foundations of emotions, attachment, communication, and self-regulation.* New York, NY: W. W. Norton.

Posner, J., Cha, J., Wang, Z., Talati, A., Warner, V., Gerber A., . . . Weissman, M. (2016). Increased default mode network connectivity in individuals at high familial risk for depression. *Neuropsychopharmacology, 41*, 1759–1767. doi:10.1038/npp.2015.342

Powers, W. T. (1973). *Behavior and the control of perception.* New York, NY: Aldine.

Qin, J., Li, R., Raes, J., Arumugam, M., Burgdorf, K. S., Manichanh, C., . . . Wang, J. (2010). A human gut microbial gene catalogue established by metagenomic sequencing. *Nature, 464*, 59–65. doi:10.1038/nature08821

Quiroga, R. Q., Reddy, L., Kreiman, G., Koch, C., & Fried, I. (2005). Invariant visual representation by single neurons in the human brain. *Nature, 435*, 1102–1107. doi:10.1038/nature03687

Ramachandran, V. S. (2011). *The tell-tale brain: Unlocking the mystery of human nature.* London, United Kingdom: Windmill Books.

Ressler, K. J., & Nemeroff, C. B. (2000). Role of serotonergic and noradrenergic systems in the pathophysiology of depression and anxiety disorders. *Depression and Anxiety, 12*(S1), 2–19.

Revlin, R. (2012). *Cognition: Theory and practice.* New York, NY: Worth.

Rhee, S. H., Pothoulakis, C., & Mayer, E. A. (2009). Principles and clinical implications of the brain–gut–enteric microbiota axis. *Nature Reviews Gastroenterology & Hepatology, 6*, 306–314. doi:10.1038/nrgastro.2009.35

Rizzolatti, G., & Arbib, M. A. (1998). Language within our grasp. *Trends in Neurosciences, 21*, 188–194.

Rosch, P. J. (2015). Why the heart is much more than a pump. In M. Dahlitz & G. Hall (Eds.), *An issue of the heart* [Special issue of *The Neuropsychotherapist*] (pp. 1–13). Brisbane, Australia: Dahlitz Media.

Rosenberg, D. R., & Keshavan, M. S. (1998). Toward a neurodevelopmental model of obsessive–compulsive disorder. *Biological Psychiatry 43*, 623–640. doi:10.1016/S0006-3223(97)00443-5

Rossouw, P. J. (2011, July). The triune brain: Implications for neuropsychotherapy. *Neuropsychotherapy News, 5*, 2–4. Retrieved from mediros.com.au/wp-content/uploads/2012/11/NPTIG-Newsletter-5.pdf

Rossouw, P. J. (Ed.). (2014). *Neuropsychotherapy: Theoretical underpinnings and clinical applications.* Brisbane, Australia: Mediros.

Rothschild, B. (2000). *The body remembers: The psychophysiology of trauma and trauma treatment.* New York, NY: W. W. Norton.

Savitz, J. B., Nugent, A. C., Bogers, W., Roiser, J. P., Bain, E. E., Neumeister, A., . . . Drevets, W. C. (2011). Habenula volume in bipolar disorder and major depressive disorder: A high-resolution magnetic resonance imaging study. *Biological Psychiatry, 69*, 336–343. doi:10.1016/j.biopsych.2010.09.027

Saxena, S., & Rauch, S. L. (2000). Functional neuroimaging and the neuroanatomy of obsessive–compulsive disorder. *Psychiatric Clinics of North America, 23*, 563–586.

Saxena, S., Gorbis, E., O'Neil, J., Baker, S. K., Mandelkern, M. A., Maidment, K. M., . . . London, E. D. (2009). Rapid effects of brief intensive cognitive-behavioral therapy on brain glucose metabolism in obsessive–compulsive disorder. *Molecular Psychiatry, 14*, 197–205. doi:10.1038/sj.mp.4002134

Schacter, D. L. (1987). Implicit memory: History and current status. *Journal of Experimental Psychology: Learning, Memory, and Cognition, 13*, 501–518. doi:10.1037/0278-7393.13.3.501

Schildkraut, J. J. (1965). The catecholamine hypothesis of affective disorders: A review of supporting evidence. *American Journal of Psychiatry, 122*, 509–522. doi:10.1176/ajp.122.5.509

Schmaal, L., Veltman, D. J., van Erp, T. G. M., Samann, P. G., Frodl, T., Jahanshad, N., . . . Hibar, D. P. (2016).

Subcortical brain alterations in major depressive disorder: Findings from the ENIGMA Major Depressive Disorder working group. *Molecular Psychiatry, 21*, 806–812. doi:10.1038/mp.2015.69

Schore, A. N. (2012). *The science of the art of psychotherapy*. New York, NY: W. W. Norton.

Shulman, G. L., Corbetta, M., Buckner, R. L., Fiez, J. A., Miezin, F. M., Raichle, M. E., & Petersen, S. E. (1997). Common blood flow changes across visual tasks: I. Increases in subcortical structures and cerebellum but not in nonvisual cortex. *Journal of Cognitive Neuroscience, 9*, 624–647. doi:10.1162/jocn.1997.9.5.624

Shulman, G. L., Fiez, J. A., Corbetta, M., Buckner, R. L., Miezin, F. M., Raichle, M. E., & Petersen, S. E. (1997). Common blood flow changes across visual tasks: II. Decreases in cerebral cortex. Journal of Cognitive Neuroscience, 9, 648–663. doi:10.1162/jocn.1997.9.5.648

Shelton, R. C., & Miller, A. H. (2010). Eating ourselves to death (and despair): The contribution of adiposity and inflammation to depression. *Progress in Neurobiology, 91*, 275–299. doi:10.1016/j.pneurobio.2010.04.004

Shepherd, A. M., Laurens, K. R., Matheson, S. L., Carr, V. J., & Green M. J. (2012). Systematic meta-review and quality assessment of the structural brain alterations in schizophrenia. *Neuroscience & Biobehavioral Reviews, 36*, 1342–1356. doi:10.1016/j.neubiorev.2011.12.015

Shimizu, E., Hashimoto, K., Okamura, N., Koike, K., Komatsu, N., Kumakiri, C., . . . Iyo, M. (2003). Alterations of serum levels of brain-derived neurotrophic factor (BDNF) in depressed patients with or without antidepressants. *Biological Psychiatry, 54*, 70–75. doi:10.1016/S0006-3223(03)00181-1

Siegel, D. J. (2007). *The mindful brain: Reflections and attunement in the cultivation of well-being*. New York, NY: W. W. Norton.

Siegel, D. J. (2012). *The developing mind: How relationships and the brain interact to shape who we are* (2nd ed.). New York, NY: Guilford Press.

Smith, E. C., & Grawe, K. (2003). What makes psychotherapy sessions productive? A new approach to bridging the gap between process research and practice. *Clinical Psychology & Psychotherapy, 10*, 275–285. doi:10.1002/cpp.377

Smith, S. M., Nichols, T. E., Vidaurre, D., Winkler, A. M., Behrens, T. E. J., Glasser, M. F., . . . Miller, K. L. (2015). A positive-negative mode of population covariation links brain connectivity, demographics and behavior. *Nature Neuroscience, 18*, 1565–1567. doi:10.1038/nn.4125

Squire, L. R. (2004). Memory systems of the brain: A brief history and current perspective. *Neurobiology of Learning and Memory, 82*, 171–177. doi:10.1016/j.nlm.2004.06.005

Stamatakis, A. M., & Stuber, G. D. (2012). Activation of lateral habenula inputs to the ventral midbrain promotes behavioral avoidance. *Nature Neuroscience, 15*, 1105–1107. doi:10.1038/nn.3145

Staum, M. S. (2003). *Labeling people: French scholars on society, race, and empire, 1815–1848*. London, United Kingdom: McGill-Queen's University Press.

Stroop, J. R. (1935). Studies of interference in serial verbal reactions. *Journal of Experimental Psychology, 18*, 643–662. doi:10.1037/h0054651.

Sudo, N., Chida, Y., Aiba, Y., Sonoda, J., Oyama, N., Yu, . . . Koga, Y. (2004). Postnatal microbial colonization programs the hypothalamic–pituitary–adrenal system for stress response in mice. *The Journal of Physiology, 558*, 263–275. doi:10.1113/jphysiol.2004.063388

Sukoff Rizzo, S. J., Neal, S. J., Hughes, Z. A., Beyna, M., Rosenzweig-Lipson, S., Moss, S. J., & Brandon, N. J. (2012). Evidence for sustained elevation of IL-6 in the CNS as a key contributor of depressive-like phenotypes. *Translational Psychiatry, 2*, e199. doi:10.1038/tp.2012.120

Sullivan, P. F., Neale, M. C., & Kendler, K. S. (2000). Genetic epidemiology of major depression: Review and meta-analysis. *The American Journal of Psychiatry, 157*, 1552–1562. doi:10.1176/appi.ajp.157.10.1552

Suomi, S. J. (1999). Attachment in rhesus monkeys. In J. Cassidy & P. R. Shaver (Eds.), *Handbook of attachment: Theory, research, and clinical applications* (pp. 181–197). New York, NY: Guilford Press.

Svob, C., Wang, Z., Weissman, M. M., Wickramaratne, P., & Posner, J. (2016). Religious and spiritual importance moderate relation between default mode network connectivity and familial risk for depression. *Neuroscience Letters, 634*, 94–97. doi:10.1016/j.neulet.2016.10.009

Tarlacı, S., & Pregnolato, M. (2016). Quantum neurophysics: From non-living matter to quantum neurobiology and psychopathology. *International Journal of Psychophysiology, 103*, 161–173. doi:10.1016/j.ijpsycho.2015.02.016

Teglasi, H., & Epstein, S. (1998). Temperament and

personality theory: The perspective of cognitive-experiential self-theory. *School Psychology Review, 27*, 534–550.

Thayer, J. F., & Lane, R. D. (2000). A model of neurovisceral integration in emotion regulation and dysregulation. *Journal of Affective Disorders, 61*, 201–216. doi:10.1016/S0165-0327(00)00338-4

The Neuropsychotherapy Institute (Producer). (2014a). Genes, neurons & glia: The wonder of the social brain [Video file]. Retrieved from http://neuropsychotherapyinstitute.com/genes-neurons-glia/

The Neuropsychotherapy Institute (Producer). (2014b). Key neurochemicals [Video file]. Retrieved from http://neuropsychotherapyinstitute.com/c07-key-neurochemicals/

Thomason, M. E., Chang, C. E., Glover, G. H., Gabrieli, J. D. E., Greicius, M. D., & Gotlib, I. H. (2008). Default-mode function and task-induced deactivation have overlapping brain substrates in children. *NeuroImage, 41*, 1493–1503. doi:10.1016/j.neuroimage.2008.03.029

Trafton, A. (2015, August 31). Possible new weapon against PTSD: Blocking a newly identified memory pathway could prevent the disorder [Web log post]. Retrieved from http://news.mit.edu/2015/blocking-memory-pathway-prevent-ptsd-0831

Trafton, A. (2017, April 6). Neuroscientists identify brain circuit necessary for memory formation [Web log post]. Retrieved from http://news.mit.edu/2017/neuroscientists-identify-brain-circuit-necessary-memory-formation-0406

Treadway, M. T., & Zald, D. H. (2011). Reconsidering anhedonia in depression: Lessons from translational neuroscience. *Neuroscience & Biobehavioral Reviews, 35*, 537–555. doi:10.1016/j.neubiorev.2010.06.006

Trzesniewski, K. H., Donnellan, M. B., & Robins, R. W. (2013). Development of self-esteem. In V. Zeigler-Hill (Ed.), *Self-esteem* (pp. 60–79). Florence, KY: Psychology Press.

Velden, M., & Wölk, C. (1987). Depicting cardiac activity over real time: A proposal for standardization. *Journal of Psychophysiology, 1*, 173–175.

Verkhratsky, A., & Butt, A. (2007). *Glial neurobiology: A textbook.* Chichester, United Kingdom: John Wiley & Sons.

Villanueva, R. (2013). Neurobiology of major depressive disorder. *Neural Plasticity, 2013*, e873278. doi:10.1155/2013/873278

Vollenweider, F. X., & Kometer, M. (2010). The neurobiology of psychedelic drugs: Implications for the treatment of mood disorders. *Nature Reviews Neuroscience, 11*, 642–651. doi:10.1038/nrn2884

Wagatsuma, A., Azami, S., Sakura, M., Hatakeyama, D., Aonuma, H., & Ito, E. (2006). De Novo synthesis of CREB in a presynaptic neuron is required for synaptic enhancement involved in memory consolidation. *Journal of Neuroscience Research, 84*, 954–960. doi:10.1002/jnr.21012

Wallace, D. J., & Hallegua, D. S. (2002). Fibromyalgia: The gastrointestinal link. *Current Pain and Headache Reports, 8*, 364–368. doi:10.1007/s11916-996-0009-z

Wallin, D. J. (2007). *Attachment in psychotherapy.* New York, NY: Guilford Press.

Washington, S. D., Gordon, E. M., Brar, J., Warburton, S., Sawyer, A. T., Wolfe, A., . . . VanMeter, J. W. (2013). Dysmaturation of the default mode network in autism. *Human Brain Mapping, 35*, 1284–1296. doi:10.1002/hbm.22252

WHO. (2016). Depression fact sheet. Retrieved from http://www.who.int/mediacentre/factsheets/fs369/en/

Wölk C., & Velden, M. (1989). Revision of the baroreceptor hypothesis on the basis of the new cardiac cycle effect. In N. W. Bond & D. A. T. Siddle (Eds.), *Psychobiology: Issues and applications* (pp. 371–379). Amsterdam, Netherlands: Elsevier.

Woo, C.-W., Koban, L., Kross, E., Lindquist, M. A., Banich, M. T., Ruzic, L., . . . Wager, T. D. (2014). Separate neural representations for physical pain and social rejection. *Nature Communications, 5*, e5380. doi:10.1038/ncomms6380

Yerys, B. E., Gordon, E. M., Abrams, D. N., Satterthwaite, T. D., Weinblatt, R., Jankowski, K. F., . . . Vaidya, C. J. (2015). Default mode network segregation and social deficits in autism spectrum disorder: Evidence from non-medicated children. *NeuroImage: Clinical, 9*, 223–232. doi:10.1016/j.nicl.2015.07.018

Zeigler-Hill, V. (Ed.). (2013). *Self-esteem.* Florence, KY: Psychology Press.

INDEX

FURTHER READING

The following books are part of the authors library and cover much of the theoretical and practical application of neuropsychotherapy for the clinician. A few of these books are detailed reference books, like *Principles of Neural Science*, some take you on a detailed journey such as McGilchrist's *The Master and His Emissary* or Kendel's *The Age of Insight,* but the majority are mostly practical clinical wisdom gleaned from neuroscience.

Arden, J. (2010). *Rewire your brain: Think your way to a better life.* Hoboken, New Jersey: John Wiley & Sons.

Arden, J. (2014). *The brain bible: How to stay vital, productive, and happy for a lifetime.* New York, NY: McGraw-Hill.

Arden, J. (2014). *Brain based therapy for anxiety - A workbook for clinicians and clients.* Eau Claire, WI: PESI Publishing.

Arden, J. (2015). Brain2brain: *Enacting client change through the persuasive power of neuroscience.* Hoboken, New Jersey: John Wiley & Sons.

Badenoch, B. (2008). *Being a brain-wise therapist: A practical guide to interpersonal neurobiology.* New York, NY: W. W. Norton & Co.

Badenoch, B. (2011). *The brain-savvy therapist's workbook: A companion to being a brain-wise therapist.* New York, NY: Norton & Co.

Brown, D. P., & Elliott, D. S. (2016). *Attachment disturbances in adults: Treatment for comprehensive repair.* New York, NY: Norton & Co.

Courtois, C. A., & Ford, J. D. (Eds.) (2014). *Treating complex traumatic stress disorders: Scientific foundations and Therapeutic Models.* New York, NY: Guilford Press.

Cozolino, L. (2008). *The healthy aging brain: Sustaining attachment, attaining wisdom.* New York, NY: Norton & Co.

Cozolino, L. (2013). *The social neuroscience of education: Optomizing attachment and learning in the classroom.* New York, NY: W. W. Norton & Co.

Cozolino, L. (2014). *The neuroscience of human relationships: Attachment and the developing social brain* (2nd ed.). New York, NY: Norton & Co.

Dahlitz, M., & Hall, G. (Eds.) (2015). *Memory Reconsolidation in psychotherapy - The neuropsychotherapist special issue.* Brisbane, Australia: Dahlitz Media.

Ecker, B., & Hulley, L. (1996). *Depth orientated brief therapy: How to be brief when you were trained to be deep - and vice versa.* San Francisco, CA: Jossey-Bass Publishers.

Ecker, B., Ticic, R. & Hulley, L. (2012). *Unlocking the emotional brain: Eliminating symptoms at their roots using memory reconsolidation.* New York, NY: Routledge.

Fisher, S. F. (2014). *Neurofeedback in the treatment of developmental trauma: Calming the fear-driven brain.* New York, NY: Norton & Co.

Fogel, A. (2009). *Body sense: The science and practice of embodied self-awareness.* New York, NY: Norton & Co.

Frewen, P., & Lanius, R. (2015). *Healing the traumatized self: Consciousness, neuroscience, treatment.* New York, NY: Norton & Co.

Gantt, S., & Badenoch, B. (Eds) (2013). *The interpersonal neurobiology of group psychotherapy and group process.* New York, NY: Norton & Co.

Grawe, K. (2007). *Neuropsychotherapy: How the neurosciences inform effective psychotherapy.* New York, NY: Psychology Press.

Hernam, J. (1992). *Trauma and recovery: The aftermath of violence - from domestic abuse to political terror.* New York, NY: Basic Books.

Hughes, D. A., & Baylin, J. (2012). *Brain-based parenting: The neuroscience of caregiving for healthy attachment.* New York, NY: Norton & Co.

Johnston, E., & Olson, L. (2015). *The feeling brain: The biology and psychology of emotions.* New York, NY: Norton & Co.

Kabat-Zinn, J. (1994). *Wherever you go there you are: Mindfulness meditation in everyday life* (10th anniversary ed.). New York, NY: Hyperion.

Kabat-Zinn, J. (2013). *Full catastrophe living: Using the wisdom of your body and mind to face stress, pain, and illness* (Revised Ed.). New York, NY: Bantam Books.

Kandel, E. R. (2006). *In search of memory: The emergence of a new science of mind.* New York, NY: W.W. Norton & Co.

Kandel, E. R. (2012). *The age of insight: The quest to understand the unconscious in art, mind, and brain - from Vienna 100 to the present.* New York, NY: Random House.

Kandel, E. R., Schwartz, J. H., Jessell, T. M., Siegelbaum, S.A., & Hudspeth, A. J. (Eds.) (2012). *Principles of Neural Science, 5th ed.* New York, NY: McGraw-Hill.

Keysers, C. (2011). *The empathic brain: How the discovery of mirror neurons changes our understanding of human nature.* Amazon Digital Services. https://www.amazon.com/Empathic-Brain-Christian-Keysers-ebook/dp/B0054S7DOO

Kosslyn, S. M., & Miller, G. W. (2013). *Top brain, bottom brain: Surprising insights into how you think.* New York, NY: Simon & Schuster.

Lambert, K. G., & Kinsley, C. H. (2004). *Clinical neuroscience: The neurobiological foundations of mental health.* New York, NY: Worth.

Lambert, K., & Kinsley, C. (2010). *Clinical neuroscience: Psychopathology and the brain (2nd ed.).* Melbourne, Australia: Oxford University Press.

Lieberman, M. D. (2013). *Social: Why our brains are wired to connect.* New York, NY: Crown.

Marks-Tarlow, T. (2012). *Clinical intuition in psychotherapy: The neurobiology of embodied response.* New York, NY: Norton & Co.

McCraty, R. (2015a). Heart-brain neurodynamics: The making of emotions. In Dahlitz, M., & Hall, G. (Eds.), *An issue of the heart: The Neuropsychotherapist special issue* (pp. 76–110). Brisbane, Australia: Dahlitz Media.

McCraty, R. (2015b). *Science of the heart: Exploring the role of the heart in human performance (Vol. 2).* Boulder Creek, CA: HeartMath Institute. Retrieved from https://www.heartmath.org/research/science-of-the-heart/

McGilchrist, I. (2009). *The master and his emissary: The divided brain and the making of the western world.* New Haven: Yale University Press.

Montgomery, A. (2013). *Neurobiology essentials for clinicians: What every therapist needs to know.* New York, NY: Norton & Co.

Ogden, P., & Fisher, J. (2015). *Sensorimotor psychotherapy: Interventions for trauma and attachment.* New York, NY: Norton & Co.

Ogden, P., Minton, K., & Pain, C. (2006). *Trauma and the body: A sensorimotor approach to psychotherapy.* New York, NY: Norton & Co.

Olson, K. (2014). *The invisible classroom: Relationships, neuroscience & mindfulness in school.* New York, NY: Norton & Co.

Panksepp, J., & Biven, L. (2012). *The archaeology of mind: Neuroevolutionary origins of human emotions.* New York, NY: W. W. Norton & Co.

Pinel, P. J., & Barnes, S. J. (2012). *Introduction to biopsychology, 9th edition.* Essex, England: Pearson Education Limited.

Porges, S. (2011). *The polyvagal theory: Neurophysiological foundations of emotions, attachment, communication, and self-regulation.* New York, NY: W. W. Norton.

Ramachandran, V. S. (2011). *The tell-tale brain: Unlocking the mystery of human nature.* London, United Kingdom: Windmill Books.

Rossouw, P. J. (Ed.) (2014). *Neuropsychotherapy: Theoretical underpinnings and clinical applications.* Brisbane, Qld: Mediros Pty Ltd.

Rothschild, B. (2000). *The body remembers: The psychophysiology of trauma and trauma treatment.* New York, NY: W. W. Norton & Co.

Rothschild, B. (2003). *The body remembers casebook: Unifying methods and models in the treatment of trauma and PTSD.* New York, NY: W. W. Norton & Co.

Scaer, R. (2005). *The trauma spectrum: Hidden wounds and human resiliency.* New York, NY: Norton & Co.

Schore, A., N. (2012). *The science of the art of psychotherapy.* New York, NY: Norton.

Siegel, D. J. (2007). *The mindful brain: Reflections and attunement in the cultivation of well-being.* New York, NY: W. W. Norton & Co.

Siegel, D. J. (2012). *The developing mind: How relationships and the brain interact to shape who we are (2nd ed.).* New York, NY: Guilford Press.

Solomon, M. F., & Siegel, D. J. (Eds.) (2003). *Healing trauma: attachment, mind, body, and brain.* New York, NY: Norton & Co.

Steele, K., Boon, S., & Van Der Hart, O. (2017). *Treating trauma-related dissociation: A practical, integrative approach.* New York, NY: Norton & Co.

Tatkin, S. (2011). *Wired for love: How understanding your partner's brain and attachment style can help you defuse conflict and build a secure relationship.* Oakland, CA: New Harbinger Publications.

Van Der Kolk, B. (2014). *The body keeps the score: Mind, brain and body in the transformation of trauma.* London, England: Allen Lane.

Verkhratsky, A., & Butt, A. (2007). *Glial neurobiology: A textbook.* Chichester, West Sussex: John Wiley & Sons Ltd.

Wilkinson, M. (2010). *Changing minds in therapy: Emotion, attachment, trauma & neurobiology.* New York, NY: Norton & Co.

PHOTO CREDITS

Bigstock.com photo credits:

I digitalista

II-III Sergey Nivens

IX Liang Zhang

1. forestpath

3. Inked Pixels

5-6. guniita

7. Cyborgwitch

11. ktsdesign

12. guniita

13. guniita

14. designua

15. designua

16. guniita

17. SFC

19-20. guniita, Eraxion

22. guniita, Eraxion

23. Eraxion

24. guniita, Eraxion

26. Eraxion

27. Sergey Nivens

28. Anna Him

30. decade3d

31. decade3d, Nerthuz

33. guniita

34. Morphart

35. Spectral-Design

36. Maria Schmitt, foxterrier2005

38. Meletver, udaix

40. Cordeschi

41. ktsdesign

42. udaix

43. udaix

45. bmfstock

46. logoboom

47. www.BillionPhotos.com

48. Kasia Bialasiewicz

49. Anna Kucherova

51. mlorenz

52. guniita

57. Ocus Focus

60. leeser

61. guniita

62. budabar

63-64. maurus

65. wiseangel

66. Dakota

67. Eraxion

69. smaglov

70. Nyul

71. Golden Brown

72. Ammentorp

73. gemenacom

75. jorgenmac

76. lightwavemedia

77. cartoon resource

78. Kurhan

79. buso23

81. Wstockstudio

82. guniita

83. Wstockstudio

84. decade3d

85. hikrcn

87. guniita

88. Kasia Bialasiewicz

89. oolulu

91. sanchairat

92. stockasso

93. Eraxion

94. Croisy

96. Eraxion

97. Eraxion, Kateryna Kon

98. Eraxion

99. dolgachov

100. Rawpixel.com

101. TitovStudio

103. ktsdesign

104. wrangler

106. Oleg Golovnev

107. Yastremska

109. Kasia Bialasiewicz

110. satariel

111. EpicStockMedia

113. alenkasm

114. alenkasm

116. igor stevanovic

117. Tatyana_Tomsickova

118. VadimGuzhva

119. Grekov

120. diego cervo

121. gstockstudio

122. Wavebreak Media Ltd

123. Wavebreak Media Ltd

124. Kasia Bialasiewicz

125. Kasia Bialasiewicz

126. Dmytro Sidelnikov

127-128. EpicStockMedia

Made in the USA
Lexington, KY
24 April 2018